ESSENTIAL ANTI-INFLAMMATORY DIET RECIPES FOR BEGINNERS

COOK YOUR WAY TO BETTER HEALTH.

CONTENTS

PREFACE

Welcome to "The Complete Anti-Inflammatory Diet Cookbook for Beginners: A Comprehensive Guide with Quick & Easy Recipes to Heal Your Immune System, Prevent Chronic Diseases, and Restore Your Body." In the hustle and bustle of our modern lives, maintaining good health and well-being has never been more important. We are bombarded by stress, processed foods, and environmental toxins that can wreak havoc on our bodies. In response to this growing health concern, the anti-inflammatory diet has emerged as a beacon of hope, offering a path to rejuvenate our immune systems, prevent chronic diseases, and restore our bodies to their natural, vibrant state.

In this book, we embark on a transformative journey through the world of anti-inflammatory eating. Whether you're a seasoned pro or just beginning to explore the concept of an anti-inflammatory diet, you'll find this comprehensive guide to be an invaluable resource. We've carefully crafted this cookbook to provide you with not only an understanding of the anti-inflammatory diet but also a treasure trove of quick and easy recipes that make it both accessible and delicious.

Your body has an incredible ability to heal itself when given the right tools. The anti-inflammatory diet equips you with these tools. By incorporating nutrient-rich, inflammation-fighting foods into your daily meals, you can take control of your health and unlock the potential for a vibrant and disease-free life.

This book will be your guide on this exciting journey. We'll explore the science behind inflammation and its role in chronic diseases, and we'll provide you with practical tips and delicious recipes to help you embrace this new way of eating. We aim to make the transition to an anti-inflammatory lifestyle as smooth as possible, ensuring that you not only understand the "why" but also the "how" of this transformative diet.

So, if you're ready to embark on a journey to wellness, join us in the pages of "The Complete Anti-Inflammatory Diet Cookbook for Beginners." Together, we will discover the healing power of food, prevent chronic diseases, and restore your body to a state of optimal health and vitality. Your path to a healthier, happier you begins right here.

CHAPTER 1
Understanding the Anti-Inflammatory Diet

Inflammation serves as a natural mechanism to initiate healing, enhancing blood circulation for a biological purpose. The interplay of the immune and vascular systems, along with various chemical mediators, orchestrates this complex process. This increased blood flow carries white blood cells and nutrients to areas of injury or infection, where they combat invading pathogens and facilitate the repair of damage. Inflammation is characterized by common signs such as discomfort, swelling, heat, and redness.

However, when inflammation becomes chronic or persistent, it can lead to various health issues. This chronic inflammation has earned a dubious reputation due to its association with several diseases, including but not limited to:

- Autoimmune diseases
- Diabetes
- Arthritic conditions
- Alzheimer's disease
- Atherosclerosis (hardening of arteries, increasing the risk of heart disease and stroke)
- Attention Deficit Disorder (ADD) and Attention Deficit Hyperactivity Disorder (ADHD)
- Inflammatory bowel disease
- Asthma and allergies
- Soft tissue swelling, often leading to pain through the irritation of nerve endings.

Enter the concept of anti-inflammatory nutrition. Recognizing that different foods are metabolized in distinct ways, this dietary approach aims to promote optimal health and healing by selecting foods that reduce inflammation. Effectively managing excessive inflammation through natural means, such as dietary choices, reduces reliance on anti-inflammatory drugs, which can have undesirable and harmful side effects without addressing the underlying issue.

Fundamental principles of an anti-inflammatory diet include:

- Prioritizing fresh fruits and vegetables, whole grains, anti-inflammatory fats, and minerals while avoiding processed foods, refined sugar, dairy products, animal protein, flavor enhancers, and food sensitivities.

Plant-based foods play a central role:

- Embrace a diverse array of fresh fruits and vegetables, rich in minerals, antioxidants, and vitamins crucial for your health.

- Certain fruits like pineapple and papaya, known for their high bromelain content, are potent natural anti-inflammatories.
- Select organic products to avoid the potentially harmful residues of herbicides and pesticides found in conventionally grown goods, some of which are genetically modified (GMOs).

For some individuals, nightshade vegetables (e.g., tomatoes, eggplants, and potatoes) may contribute to inflammation, and their consumption should be limited or avoided.

When it comes to fats:

- Opt for healthy anti-inflammatory fats like coconut oil, olive oil, avocados, and fatty fish, all of which promote well-being.
- Limit or avoid saturated fats, trans-fats, hydrogenated oils, and dairy fats.

Regarding meat consumption:

- Animal proteins, particularly beef, pork, and farmed eggs, should be limited or avoided due to their potential to induce inflammation.
- Opt for sources like fish, free-range poultry, organic lamb, and omega-3 enriched eggs.

Dairy products should be limited or avoided due to the loss of lactase enzymes with age, contributing to lactose intolerance and inflammation.

When it comes to grains:

- Prioritize whole grains over refined grains to preserve essential nutrients and fiber.
- Whole grains also provide complex carbohydrates, which help regulate blood sugar and prevent inflammation, unlike simple sugars.

Nuts and seeds can be included in your diet:

- Enjoy varieties like almonds, sesame seeds, walnuts, flaxseeds, and pumpkin seeds.
- Be cautious if you have specific allergies to certain nuts.

In terms of beverages:

- Consume clean, filtered water and herbal teas, avoiding sugary sodas, fruit juices with added sugars, and excessive dairy.

Spices like oregano, turmeric, ginger, rosemary, cinnamon, and garlic can be beneficial for reducing inflammation. These spices contain bioflavonoids and polyphenols that combat inflammation and neutralize disease-causing free radicals.

Choose natural sweeteners:

- Stevia, maple syrup, molasses, and honey are healthier alternatives compared to refined sugar.
- Avoid refined sugar, high fructose corn syrup, and artificial sweeteners, which can promote inflammation.

Consider incorporating fermented foods into your diet, such as sauerkraut, kimchi, and miso soup. These foods, rich in probiotics, help maintain a healthy gut microbiota, reducing inflammation and improving immune function.

Eliminate processed foods, artificial colors, artificial flavors, and preservatives. If you have known food sensitivities or allergies that contribute to inflammation, avoid those as well. Common culprits include wheat (gluten), corn, soy, and dairy.

In essence, the power of good health lies in our natural choices. With numerous anti-inflammatory nutritional recipes available, you can easily navigate the world of anti-inflammatory eating for a healthier, happier life.

Who Can Benefit from the Anti-Inflammatory Diet.

Were you aware that inflammation lies at the root of numerous chronic diseases such as arthritis, obesity, heart disease, diabetes, and even cancer? Yes, it's true. A significant portion of chronic diseases arises from a lifestyle that encourages the consumption of the wrong foods in excessive amounts and at inappropriate times. These dietary choices set in motion various processes within your body, giving rise to inflammation from multiple sources. Moreover, many of us possess genetic predispositions that lead to heightened inflammation when confronted with common irritants such as smoke, chemicals, and dietary imbalances. Some individuals experience such excessive inflammation that they develop autoimmune diseases like multiple sclerosis (MS), lupus, rheumatoid arthritis, colitis, and psoriasis.

So, how do poor food choices trigger inflammation? Among the worst culprits are frozen and highly processed foods, as well as fast food, which happen to be some of the most readily available food options. These convenience foods are designed for shelf-life and taste enhancement, achieved by incorporating trans-fats – a type of unhealthy fat – that originates from the hydrogenation of saturated fats. This transformed fat, chemically distinct from naturally occurring fats, initiates a chain reaction of chemicals known as cytokines in your body tissues. Cytokines are molecules that drive inflammation in your body.

Another source of inflammatory foods includes those high in refined sugars. Pastries like cakes, doughnuts, and cookies are examples of easily digested foods that release substantial amounts of glucose into your bloodstream. This rapid glucose influx triggers elevated blood sugar levels, prompting your body to release an insulin surge to restore balance. Unfortunately, this insulin surge, combined with high blood glucose levels, contributes to the production of cytokines and other inflammatory molecules in your body. Moreover, every glucose spike signals your body to store fat, which, in turn, releases the same inflammatory molecules and cytokines.

Refined grains, which lack fiber and essential nutrients, also have inflammation-inducing properties. A whole grain consists of glucose molecules encapsulated within a fibrous coating, which slows down glucose absorption and release. However, when this fibrous coating is removed, as in the case of refined grains, the glucose molecules are easily digested and absorbed into your body, inciting the inflammatory cascade.

In some individuals, certain grains, such as oats, wheat, rye, and barley, contain a protein called gluten. Gluten is particularly harmful to people with genetic sensitivities to gluten absorption. Symptoms in such individuals can range from discomfort, flushing, diarrhea, and malnutrition to mild nausea and energy deficiency. Managing this type of inflammation often involves eliminating these specific grains from the diet.

So, what exactly is an anti-inflammatory diet? Typically, it comprises fresh, whole foods that lack inflammatory elements and are rich in molecules that actively counter inflammation in the body. Most fruits and vegetables contain phytonutrients, which owe their colorful appearance and carry both antioxidant and anti-inflammatory properties. These compounds neutralize oxidative stress, a significant source of inflammation in the body. Healthy fats found in fatty fish, flax seeds, nuts, and cooking oils like olive oil and canola oil can also reduce inflammation. Moreover, various vitamins and minerals abundant in fresh, whole foods, such as vitamins A, C, D, E, zinc, selenium, and copper, neutralize oxidative stress and dampen inflammation.

The first step in adopting an anti-inflammatory diet involves avoiding fast food and processed food. The next step is to reduce the consumption of foods containing refined sugars and processed grains. The core of the anti-inflammatory diet revolves around a generous daily intake of fresh fruits and vegetables, along with moderate portions of whole grains, lean protein, and healthy fats found in fish, seeds, and nuts. The final step, specifically for individuals with sensitivities, often involves reducing or eliminating gluten-containing grains.

Who can benefit from an anti-inflammatory diet? Anyone suffering from inflammatory disorders like autoimmune conditions (such as lupus, multiple sclerosis, rheumatoid arthritis, colitis) or allergic conditions (gastrointestinal issues, eczema) can certainly find relief with an anti-inflammatory diet. Most people dealing with chronic pain, be it headaches, neck pain, back pain, knee pain, muscle pain, or joint pain, are experiencing inflammation and can benefit from this dietary approach. Conditions like irritable bowel syndrome and common digestive problems like acid reflux tend to improve with an anti-inflammatory diet. Importantly, individuals with chronic degenerative conditions such as diabetes, arthritis, obesity, cardiovascular diseases, and even cancer can derive substantial benefits from this diet. Lastly, anyone interested in preventive health and optimal well-being will find that adopting an anti-inflammatory diet not only guards against illness and promotes overall health but also contributes to youthful longevity.

Incorporate healthy eating habits and keep inflammation at bay – this powerful way of eating holds benefits for individuals of all ages, from children to the elderly.

Were you aware that inflammation lies at the root of numerous chronic diseases such as arthritis, obesity, heart disease, diabetes, and even cancer? Yes, it's true. A significant portion of chronic diseases arises from a lifestyle that encourages the consumption of the wrong foods in excessive amounts and at inappropriate times. These dietary choices set in motion various processes within your body, giving rise to inflammation from multiple sources. Moreover, many of us possess genetic predispositions that lead to heightened inflammation when confronted with common irritants such as smoke, chemicals, and dietary imbalances. Some individuals experience such excessive inflammation that they develop autoimmune diseases like multiple sclerosis (MS), lupus, rheumatoid arthritis, colitis, and psoriasis.

So, how do poor food choices trigger inflammation? Among the worst culprits are frozen and highly processed foods, as well as fast food, which happen to be some of the most readily available food options. These convenience foods are designed for shelf-life and taste enhancement, achieved by incorporating trans-fats – a type of unhealthy fat – that originates from the hydrogenation of saturated fats. This transformed fat, chemically distinct from naturally occurring fats, initiates a chain reaction of chemicals known as cytokines in your body tissues. Cytokines are molecules that drive inflammation in your body.

Another source of inflammatory foods includes those high in refined sugars. Pastries like cakes, doughnuts, and cookies are examples of easily digested foods that release substantial amounts of glucose into your bloodstream. This rapid glucose influx triggers elevated blood sugar levels, prompting your body to release an insulin surge to restore balance. Unfortunately, this insulin surge, combined with high blood glucose levels, contributes to the production of cytokines and other inflammatory molecules in your body. Moreover, every glucose spike signals your body to store fat, which, in turn, releases the same inflammatory molecules and cytokines.

Refined grains, which lack fiber and essential nutrients, also have inflammation-inducing properties. A whole grain consists of glucose molecules encapsulated within a fibrous coating, which slows down glucose absorption and release. However, when this fibrous coating is removed, as in the case of refined grains, the glucose molecules are easily digested and absorbed into your body, inciting the inflammatory cascade.

In some individuals, certain grains, such as oats, wheat, rye, and barley, contain a protein called gluten. Gluten is particularly harmful to people with genetic sensitivities to gluten absorption. Symptoms in such individuals can range from discomfort, flushing, diarrhea, and malnutrition to mild nausea and energy deficiency. Managing this type of inflammation often involves eliminating these specific grains from the diet.

So, what exactly is an anti-inflammatory diet? Typically, it comprises fresh, whole foods that lack inflammatory elements and are rich in molecules that actively counter inflammation in the body. Most fruits and vegetables contain phytonutrients, which owe their colorful appearance and carry both antioxidant and anti-inflammatory properties. These compounds neutralize oxidative stress, a significant source of inflammation in the body. Healthy fats found in fatty fish, flax seeds, nuts, and cooking oils like olive oil and canola oil can also reduce inflammation. Moreover, various vitamins and minerals abundant in fresh, whole foods, such as vitamins A, C, D, E, zinc, selenium, and copper, neutralize oxidative stress and dampen inflammation.

The first step in adopting an anti-inflammatory diet involves avoiding fast food and processed food. The next step is to reduce the consumption of foods containing refined sugars and processed grains. The core of the anti-inflammatory diet revolves around a generous daily intake of fresh fruits and vegetables, along with moderate portions of whole grains, lean protein, and healthy fats found in fish, seeds, and nuts. The final step, specifically for individuals with sensitivities, often involves reducing or eliminating gluten-containing grains.

Who can benefit from an anti-inflammatory diet? Anyone suffering from inflammatory disorders like autoimmune conditions (such as lupus, multiple sclerosis, rheumatoid arthritis, colitis) or allergic conditions (gastrointestinal issues, eczema) can certainly find relief with an anti-inflammatory diet. Most people dealing with chronic pain, be it headaches, neck pain, back pain, knee pain, muscle pain, or joint pain, are experiencing inflammation and can benefit from this dietary approach. Conditions like irritable bowel syndrome and common digestive problems like acid reflux tend to improve with an anti-inflammatory diet. Importantly, individuals with chronic degenerative conditions such as diabetes, arthritis, obesity, cardiovascular diseases, and even cancer can derive substantial benefits from this diet. Lastly, anyone interested in preventive health and optimal well-being will find that adopting an anti-inflammatory diet not only guards against illness and promotes overall health but also contributes to youthful longevity.

Incorporate healthy eating habits and keep inflammation at bay – this powerful way of eating holds benefits for individuals of all ages, from children to the elderly

The Alkaline Anti-inflammatory Diet.

Our diet presents one of the most effective ways to maintain good health, alleviate chronic pain, manage a healthy weight, and promote a long and vibrant life. Regrettably, many of us have received inaccurate information regarding what, how, and when to eat. To start, let's delve into a bit of human history. For much of the history of humanity on this planet, we were nomadic. We roamed the Earth in search of large animals to hunt and eat. Alternatively, people herded animals like sheep, goats, and other livestock, which necessitated movement to find ample pastures. Our ancestors didn't consume excessive amounts of fat and meat; they primarily gathered fruits and only modest amounts of grains. Starchy carbohydrates, such as pasta, cereals, bread, and other grains, were scarcely present in their diet. It was only about 5,000 years ago, with the advent of farming in ancient Egypt, that people began consuming significant quantities of starchy carbohydrates.

Now, let's introduce some basic biochemistry that's easy to grasp. Most of us are familiar with fish oil and its crucial omega-3 fatty acids. However, the significance of another type of oil, omega-6 fatty acids, often goes unnoticed. Our forebears, who maintained a diet low in starchy carbohydrates and led a nomadic lifestyle, had a diet that consisted of approximately equal amounts of omega-3 and omega-6 fatty acids, resulting in a balanced 1:1 ratio. This ratio is ideal for the body, making it more alkaline than acidic, with higher alkalinity being better for overall health.

However, if we become imbalanced in our intake of omega-3 and omega-6 fatty acids, our bodies tend to become more acidic and inflamed. This inflammation contributes to chronic pain, weight gain, and lifestyle-related diseases such as diabetes, cardiovascular issues, arthritis, and other contemporary health concerns. High consumption of carbohydrates like wheat, corn, and rice is often linked to an overabundance of omega-6 fatty acids, creating a substantial imbalance, with ratios like 1:10 or even higher in favor of omega-6 fatty acids. For instance, consider that potato chips can have a staggering ratio of 1:60 in favor of omega-6 over omega-3 fatty acids.

Inadequate balance in omega oils induced by excessive carbohydrate consumption results in systemic inflammation throughout the body. Conversely, a diet low in carbohydrates promotes a 1:1 ratio of fatty acids, making the body more alkaline and efficient.

To adopt an alkaline anti-inflammatory diet, reducing the intake of starchy carbohydrates is key. By limiting one's consumption to 100-200 grams of grain products per day, individuals can make a significant shift toward a healthier lifestyle. This diet should predominantly feature a substantial quantity of vegetables and a diverse range of protein and fat sources, including meats, eggs, nuts, and fish. Conversely, sugary foods like cookies, candies, sodas, sports drinks, and cakes should be minimized in this diet.

It's important to note that this diet need not be overly strict. Many individuals with a balanced metabolism can incorporate a "cheat day" or two each week, where they may consume 100-200 grams of starchy carbohydrates and enjoy some sweet treats.

While not all health professionals or nutritionists may adhere to the specifics outlined here, numerous books and medical practitioners are associated with this dietary approach. Examples include the Paleolithic Diet, South Beach Diet, Keto Diet, and Mediterranean diet. Seeking guidance from experts who support this dietary strategy is advisable.

Many individuals who adopt an alkaline anti-inflammatory diet experience noticeable improvements in their health within a reasonable time frame. Some report achieving a desirable weight within a year, alleviating back pain, boosting energy levels, and experiencing better sleep. Although the mainstream may not yet fully embrace the alkaline anti-inflammatory diet, there is a wealth of empirical and anecdotal evidence to explore this way of life.

Embracing an anti-inflammatory diet not only allows individuals to feel fantastic by reducing the consumption of pro-inflammatory foods, but it also helps alleviate discomfort and stress on joints and organs that result from the removal of these foods from the diet. Moreover, the risk of weight gain decreases when one adopts this diet. Additionally, by minimizing other sources of inflammation in the body, the anti-inflammatory diet helps mitigate various conditions, including hypertension, arthritis, fibromyalgia, Alzheimer's disease, chronic fatigue syndrome, chronic pain, asthma, cancer, acne, diabetes, heart disease, and depression. This is just a condensed list, as there are numerous other inflammatory conditions.

In summary, the less inflammatory foods we consume, the less inflammation our bodies experience. Pro-inflammatory foods primarily consist of modern crops, hydrogenated oils, refined sugars, seed oils, and vegetable oils. Although these foods have been around for a relatively short time, the rates of obesity and disease continue to rise. Human genetics are more aligned with the consumption of fruits, nuts, vegetables, fish, and meat, rather than foods associated with chronic diseases.

So, why are grains particularly problematic? Grains contain a protein called gluten, which is the primary culprit behind many digestive disorders, including celiac disease and frequent headaches. Grains also contain a sugar protein called lectins, which have been shown to induce digestive inflammation. Furthermore, grains contain phytic acid, which is known to reduce the absorption of calcium, iron, magnesium, and zinc in the body. Lastly, grains contain high levels of biochemically fatty acids known as omega-6 fatty acids, which contribute to inflammation. Conversely, fresh fish and green vegetables contain omega-3 fatty acids, which have anti-inflammatory properties.

To follow an anti-inflammatory diet, one should consume foods known for their anti-inflammatory properties. This includes all fruits, either raw or lightly cooked, delicious red pumpkins, eggs rich in omega-3 fatty acids, unprocessed grains, and spices like turmeric, ginger, and garlic. Healthy fats, such as organic coconut oil, butter, and extra virgin olive oil, are also essential components of this diet. Incorporate fresh fish while avoiding farmed varieties, and include protein sources like chicken, beef, and grass-fed eggs. Additionally, wild game such as elk and deer can be a part of this diet. Opt for beverages like water, red wine, organic green tea, and stout beer.

Exploring the Advantages of an Anti-Inflammatory Diet.

Inflammation is poised to be the next major breakthrough in medicine. Individuals dealing with obesity often experience inflammatory issues. This body inflammation is closely linked to conditions like diabetes, arthritis, and asthma, not to mention its association with heart diseases and certain types of cancer. Adopting an anti-inflammatory diet can rapidly enhance one's well-being, providing immediate benefits and long-term health improvements.

To begin an anti-inflammatory diet, it's essential to consider how food affects the body. Meat is a valuable source of essential nutrients and vitamins necessary for survival. The concept of eating to live rather than living to eat is a powerful motivator, especially for those seeking weight loss. However, this perspective should be embraced beyond just shedding a few pounds. Some foods are rich in antioxidants and natural anti-inflammatory compounds that can mitigate the body's inflammatory response, forming the foundation of the anti-inflammatory diet.

The role of omega-3 and other fatty acids is crucial. Many foods contain various types of oils that are rich in fatty acids. Fish like sardines and salmon stand out as the best natural sources. However, Western diets often contain an abundance of omega-6 fatty acids compared to omega-3s. Foods like chicken, turkey, eggs, nuts, and vegetable oils are rich in omega-6 fatty acids. A balanced intake of both omega-3 and omega-6 fatty acids is essential for optimal health and anti-inflammatory effects. The Western diet, in contrast, frequently features an omega-6 to omega-3 ratio of 10:1 or even 30:1, while the ideal balance is closer to 4:1, favoring omega-6 fatty acids. Increasing the intake of omega-3 fatty acids through sources like fish oils, kiwis, black raspberries, assorted nuts, and particularly flaxseeds can help reduce body inflammation and its associated health implications.

Another simple adjustment to minimize inflammation is reducing the consumption of fatty meats. Among all meats, red meat is particularly problematic for those prone to inflammation. Opting for leaner cuts or lean substitutes like bison and venison is a wise choice. Additionally, grass-fed beef has less unfavorable properties for the body. Meats like chicken, turkey, and soy-based products such as tofu and soy milk are excellent alternatives to decrease inflammation. While some of these meats may contain more omega-6 fatty acids, you can address this fatty acid imbalance by cooking these meats in olive oil or adding flaxseed oil to the final dish to enhance the intake of omega-3s and alleviate inflammation.

Ridding your diet of refined carbohydrates is another key step in reducing inflammation. Refined carbohydrates have minimal nutritional value and should be replaced with whole-grain alternatives. Almost all flour is wheat-based, but refined flour is devoid of the natural grains and is typically bleached, leaving behind empty calories that contribute to body inflammation. Simply swapping out white bread for whole-grain bread and white flour for unbleached whole wheat flour can make a significant difference in how your body responds to your diet.

An essential aspect of an anti-inflammatory diet is breakfast. Your kitchen has the potential to serve as a hub for healing and nourishing your body. A natural anti-inflammatory breakfast can energize you and provide an excellent start to your day. Interested? Great! Let's explore one of the most remarkable culinary innovations of the last century – the versatile blender. Unlike juicers that remove valuable fiber, or food processors that essentially act as knives and spoons, the Hamilton Shake method takes a simple, cost-effective approach. Here's how it works:

The Anti-Inflammatory Food Ingredients:
- Begin by chopping up a pear (or use apple, grapefruit, mango, papaya, or kiwi, depending on your preference) into chunks and place it in the blender.
- Add half a cup of a mixture that includes sunflower, sesame, flax, and oat. This blend provides essential fatty acids (omega-3), protein, and all the fiber of whole grains. Mix this mixture and store it in a large container in your refrigerator.
- Incorporate dark berries such as blueberries and blackberries. These berries are rich in antioxidants called flavonoids, which are as beneficial as exotic Amazonian options but more readily available and budget-friendly. Dark berries also freeze well for convenience.

The Mega Extras:
- Add turmeric, a powerful natural anti-inflammatory spice. Fresh burdock root is an excellent addition for cleansing the liver and blood.
- If nettles are in season, consider foraging them in the wild. Mixing them in neutralizes the sting and unlocks natural minerals and anti-inflammatory effects while reducing allergies.
- You can also include chopped raw carrots or celery for added nutritional value.

Now, here's the key – adjust everything else to your taste and mood. Your creativity and growing knowledge are the only limitations. Play around with ingredients. By doing so, you'll save a significant amount on vitamins and supplements. Add water and blend the ingredients until you achieve your desired consistency, either cold or warm water (or even almond milk) to suit your taste. If you have an excess, save it for later use.

This concoction is not only packed with nutrients but also serves as an excellent delivery system for an array of nutrients and medicinal herbs. It's a versatile option for breakfast or any other meal of the day, offering a blend of flavor and nutrition to support overall well-being.

Overcoming Common Challenges on an Anti-Inflammatory Diet

Everyone aspires to improve their well-being and embrace a healthier lifestyle. Transitioning from a traditional Western diet to an anti-inflammatory diet is one of the simplest and most effective ways to achieve this goal. However, it's important to recognize that while the concept is straightforward, the actual practice of making these dietary changes can be challenging, as it requires a shift in eating habits and choices.

Fast Food and Inflammation: Fast food poses a significant obstacle to adopting an anti-inflammatory diet. These types of foods, laden with high levels of fat, have been shown to increase inflammation within the body approximately three to four hours after consumption. Notably, consuming an equivalent number of calories from fresh vegetables, fruits, and lean meats does not have the same inflammatory effect. Fast food consumption can also lead to a 175% increase in free radicals, which are molecules that contribute to inflammation-related health issues.

The Alternative – A Substitutive Anti-Inflammatory Diet: An excellent alternative to fast food lies in adopting a substitute anti-inflammatory diet. Take, for example, the classic McDonald's Big Mac. This iconic sandwich can be transformed into a healthier version using lean turkey and a whole-grain bun. By substituting the traditional "special sauce" with lower-carb ketchup, mayonnaise, olive oil, and sugar-free options, you create a flavorful alternative with significantly reduced fat content.

Red Meat, Dairy, and Inflammation: For quite some time, scientific research has pointed to a connection between red meat consumption and certain types of cancer. However, the link to inflammation is relatively recent. It appears that certain chemical elements in red meat and dairy products can trigger an immune response, leading to inflammation when the body mistakenly identifies these components as foreign substances. For instance, daily consumption of red meat along with 2 to 3 cups of milk could result in a state of chronic inflammation over time, potentially leading to health complications.

Choosing Lean Proteins: Incorporating lean meats, beef, and fish into your diet is part of a balanced approach. While beef is an excellent source of iron, it's essential to opt for the leanest cuts for better health. Lean proteins and beans are healthier meat choices that help minimize inflammation.

Trans Fats and Inflammation: Trans-fatty acids are often considered a hidden source of body inflammation. Although some people have a basic understanding of these fats, few grasp their full impact on the body. Trans fats are prevalent in fast food, baked goods, pre-packaged foods, and margarine. Their intake is associated with increased risks of coronary artery disease, insulin resistance, diabetes, and heart failure. Abnormally high levels of lipids in the body also elevate the risk of stroke. It's worth noting that while some foods claim to be "trans-fat-free," they may contain up to 0.5 grams of trans fats per serving, adhering to labeling regulations.

The Choice – Opting for Natural Fats: Choosing natural fats such as whole butter and olive oil, which are free of trans fats, is a positive step in an anti-inflammatory diet. When it comes to foods cooked in trans fats, there is no alternative but to eliminate them from your diet entirely. Many individuals prefer to follow an anti-inflammatory diet by preparing their own "fast foods" at home using healthier ingredients and snacks.

CHAPTER 2
Weekly Meal Plan Featuring Slow Cooked Recipes

Week One Meal Plan

DAY ONE

BREAKFAST - Slow-Cooker Southwest Quinoa Bowls
This taco-bowl-style dish is sure to please both adults and children. Allowing it to sit for 10 minutes helps the cheese meld with the quinoa, adding a delightful richness. If you can't find Cheddar-Jack cheese, feel free to substitute with Sharp Cheddar or Monterey Jack. Garnish with lime wedges, fresh cilantro, and extra cheese if desired.

Ingredients:
- 1 yellow onion (about 8 ounces), diced
- 1 tablespoon olive oil
- 1 ripe avocado, cubed
- 1 teaspoon ground cumin
- 1 red bell pepper (about 8 ounces), diced
- 3 garlic cloves, minced (approximately 1 tablespoon)
- ¾ teaspoon kosher salt
- 1 (15-ounce) can no-salt-added black beans, drained and rinsed
- 1 teaspoon ancho chili powder
- 1 (14.5-ounce) can fire-roasted diced tomatoes
- Frozen corn kernels (from 1 ear) or 1 cup fresh
- 2 cups water
- 1 cup uncooked quinoa, rinsed
- ¼ cup chopped fresh cilantro
- 4 ounces Cheddar-Jack cheese blend, shredded (about 1 cup)

Directions:
1. Heat the olive oil in a large saucepan over medium-high heat. Add the diced onions and bell pepper, and cook, stirring constantly, for four to five minutes until they become tender. Add the garlic, cumin, and chili powder, cooking and stirring for an additional minute.
2. In a slow cooker, combine the onion mixture, corn, black beans, water, tomatoes, quinoa, and salt. Cover and cook on medium heat for 4 to 5 hours until the quinoa is tender and most of the liquid is absorbed.

3. Add the cilantro to the slow cooker and mix well. Sprinkle the shredded cheese over the quinoa mixture, cover, and let it sit for about 10 minutes until the cheese melts. Divide the mixture into six bowls and top with cubed avocado.

Nutrition Facts: Serving Size: About 1 Cup
- Calories: 364
- Carbohydrates: 44g (14% Daily Value)
- Protein: 15g (30% DV)
- Sugars: 7g
- Dietary Fiber: 10g (40% DV)
- Fat: 16g (25% DV)
- Saturated Fat: 5g (25% DV)
- Sodium: 536mg (21% DV)
- Vitamin A: <1IU
- Vitamin C: <1mg (2% DV)
- Calcium: <1mg
- Iron: <1mg (6% DV)
- Potassium: <1mg
- Thiamin: <1mg (100% DV)

LUNCH - Italian Wedding Soup

This Italian wedding soup recipe is the epitome of Italian comfort food, and it offers numerous variations. You can substitute the kale or escarole with chard, chicory, or any other leafy greens and use any leftover cooked white beans (or canned) in this healthy Italian wedding soup recipe.

Ingredients:
- 1 pound ground turkey breast
- ¼ teaspoon salt
- ½ cup dry white wine
- 1 large egg, lightly beaten
- 1 cup fresh whole-wheat breadcrumbs
- ¼ cup finely chopped fresh parsley
- 1 tablespoon Worcestershire sauce
- 2 cloves garlic, minced
- ½ teaspoon crushed fennel seeds
- ½ teaspoon freshly ground pepper
- 2 teaspoons extra-virgin olive oil
- Soup

- 1 tablespoon extra-virgin olive oil
- 1 cup chopped carrots (2 medium)
- 1 cup chopped onion (1 medium)
- 4 cups chopped cabbage (about ½ small head)
- 1 cup chopped celery (2 medium stalks)
- 1 (15-ounce) can white beans, rinsed
- 8 cups coarsely chopped escarole or thinly sliced kale leaves (about one bunch)
- 8 cups low-sodium chicken broth
- ½ cup freshly grated Romano cheese

Directions:
1. In a large bowl, combine ground turkey with breadcrumbs, Worcestershire sauce, egg, garlic, parsley, fennel seeds, pepper, and salt. Refrigerate for 10 minutes to firm up. Shape the mixture into 32 (1-inch) meatballs (approximately 1 tablespoon each) with damp hands.
2. Heat 2 teaspoons of oil in a non-stick skillet over medium heat. Cook the meatballs, turning them every few minutes, for 7-9 minutes or until they are browned on all sides. Remove from heat and add the white wine to deglaze the pan, scraping up the browned bits. Remove from heat.
3. For the soup, heat 1 tablespoon of oil in a soup pot or Dutch oven over medium heat. Add the chopped onion, carrots, and celery and cook, stirring for 7 to 9 minutes until the onion is translucent. Add cabbage and cook, stirring for an additional 5 minutes. Stir in the broth, white beans, escarole, meatballs, and any accumulated juices. Bring the soup to a boil, then reduce the heat and let it simmer for 20 to 25 minutes, stirring occasionally, until the vegetables become tender. Top each serving with 1 tablespoon of grated cheese.

Nutrition Facts: Serving Size: About 1 3/4 Cups with 4 Meatballs
- Protein: 23.9g (48% Daily Value)
- Calories: 283.7
- Carbohydrates: 23.5g (8% DV)
- Sugars: 4.6g
- Dietary Fiber: 6.3g (25% DV)
- Fat: 11.1g (17% DV)
- Saturated Fat: 3.5g (18% DV)
- Vitamin C: 21.9mg (37% DV)
- Vitamin A: 4130.1IU (83% DV)
- Folate: 141.5mcg (35% DV)
- Iron: 3.3mg (18% DV)

- Calcium: 205.7mg (21% DV)
- Magnesium: 33.3mg (12% DV)
- Sodium: 522.5mg (21% DV)
- Potassium: 869.9mg (24% DV)
- Thiamin: 0.1mg (14% DV)

Exchanges:
- 1 1/2 Vegetable
- 2 Medium-Fat Meat
- 1/2 Starch
- 1/2 Lean Meat
- 1/2 Fat

DINNER - Chicken and Farro Herb Salad

This healthy chicken salad recipe makes for an excellent potluck dish or a nutritious dinner, featuring an abundance of fresh herbs, arugula, olives, and farro. While farro imparts a sweet flavor and hearty texture, other grains such as Freekeh, Bulgur, or couscous can be equally delightful choices.

Ingredients: Red-Wine Vinaigrette
- ⅓ cup red-wine vinegar
- ½ cup extra-virgin olive oil
- 1 ½ tablespoons Dijon mustard
- ¾ teaspoon kosher salt
- 1 small clove garlic, minced
- ½ teaspoon ground pepper

Salad
- 3 cups water
- 1 ½ pounds boneless, skinless chicken breast, trimmed
- 1 cup farro
- ½ teaspoon kosher salt
- ¼ teaspoon ground pepper
- 1 cup diced carrots
- 1 fennel bulb, cored and chopped
- 1 cup chopped seeded English cucumber
- ¼ cup chopped flat-leaf parsley
- ½ cup finely chopped red onion
- ¼ cup fresh basil, very thinly sliced
- 2 cups arugula, tough stems removed, coarsely chopped

- ¼ cup fresh mint, very thinly sliced
- ¼ cup oil-cured black olives, sliced

Directions:
1. **Vinaigrette:** In a medium bowl, whisk together red-wine vinegar, garlic, Dijon mustard, 3/4 teaspoon salt, and 1/2 teaspoon pepper. Gradually whisk in the olive oil.
2. **Salad:** In a medium saucepan, bring 3 cups of water to a boil. Add the farro, reduce the heat to low, cover, and cook for 15 to 25 minutes or until it's tender. Drain the cooked farro and transfer it to a large bowl.
3. Toss the soft farro with 1/3 cup of the vinaigrette.
4. Preheat the grill to medium-high.
5. Sprinkle the chicken with salt and pepper. Brush the grill rack with oil and grill the chicken, turning occasionally, for 12 to 16 minutes or until it's cooked through. Let the chicken cool for 5 minutes and then slice it.
6. Stir in the fennel, cucumber, carrots, red onion, basil, parsley, and mint into the farro. Add one-third cup of vinaigrette and mix well.
7. Just before serving, toss the arugula into the farro mixture. Serve the salad with the grilled chicken and olives, along with the remaining vinaigrette.

Nutrition Facts: Serving Size: 1 1/3 Cups Salad & 3 Oz. Chicken
- Exchanges: 1 1/2 Vegetable
- 1 1/2 Starch
- 3 Lean Meat
- 4 Fat
- Calories: 458.8
- Carbohydrates: 31.9g (10% Daily Value)
- Protein: 28.2g (56% DV)
- Sugars: 4.8g
- Dietary Fiber: 5.3g (21% DV)
- Fat: 24.5g (38% DV)
- Saturated Fat: 3.7g (19% DV)
- Vitamin C: 12.7mg (21% DV)
- Vitamin A: 4562.4IU (91% DV)
- Folate: 141.5mcg (35% DV)
- Iron: 2.7mg (15% DV)
- Calcium: 205.7mg (21% DV)
- Magnesium: 33.3mg (12% DV)
- Sodium: 512.6mg (21% DV)
- Thiamin: 0.1mg (9% DV)

DAY THREE
BREAKFAST

Italian Roasted Pork Tenderloin with Quinoa and Veggies
For a delightful taste in this straightforward roasted pork tenderloin dish, marinate the pork the night before or in the morning before work. When you return home, you'll only need to roast the pork and vegetables and prepare the quinoa for a simple and safe dinner. This recipe yields extra quinoa, which can be used as the foundation for quick lunches, salads, or stir-fries later in the week.

Ingredients: Italian Dressing
- ¾ cup red-wine vinegar
- 1 ½ tablespoons sugar
- 5 tablespoons water
- 1 ¾ cups extra-virgin olive oil
- 1 large garlic clove
- 1 tablespoon Dijon mustard
- 2 teaspoons dried basil
- ½ teaspoon salt
- 2 teaspoons dried oregano
- ½ teaspoon ground pepper

Pork and Vegetables
- 1-pound pork tenderloin
- 2 medium parsnips
- 3 tablespoons extra-virgin olive oil, divided
- 4 medium carrots
- 1 medium broccoli crown
- 4 tablespoons balsamic glaze
- 2 teaspoons Italian seasoning
- 1 ½ teaspoons salt, divided

Quinoa
- ¼ teaspoon salt
- 3 cups low-sodium chicken broth
- 1 ½ cups quinoa
- 1 tablespoon extra-virgin olive oil

Directions:

1. **Dressing:** In a blender, combine vinegar, basil, water, mustard, sugar, garlic, oregano, salt, and pepper. Blend until smooth. Gradually add olive oil and blend until creamy (reserve 1/4 cup plus two tablespoons for later, and refrigerate the remaining dressing for up to one week).
2. **Cooking Pork and Vegetables:** Place pork and 1/4 cup of the dressing in a resealable plastic bag. Seal and refrigerate for 4 to 24 hours. Preheat the oven to 425°F, with racks in the lower and upper thirds.
3. **Prepare Vegetables:** Peel and cut parsnips and carrots into 1-inch pieces. Cut broccoli into large florets. Toss these veggies with Italian seasoning, 1/2 teaspoon salt, and the remaining 2 tablespoons of dressing. Spread them on a large rimmed baking sheet.
4. **Roast Pork:** Remove pork from the marinade and pat it dry. Sprinkle with the remaining 1/4 teaspoon of salt and pepper. Heat one tablespoon of oil in a large ovenproof skillet and brown the pork for 3 to 5 minutes. Transfer pork to the upper oven rack, place the vegetables on the lower rack, and roast the pork until it reaches 145°F, which takes about 20 minutes. Roast the vegetables for about 20 to 25 minutes, stirring occasionally.
5. **Prepare Quinoa:** Combine quinoa, chicken broth, 1/4 teaspoon salt, and one tablespoon of oil in a large saucepan. Bring to a boil, then simmer until the liquid is absorbed and the grains are tender, about 15-20 minutes. Cover and let it sit for 5 minutes.
6. **Rest and Serve:** Let the pork rest for 5 minutes on a cutting board, then slice it. Toss the remaining two tablespoons of dressing with the vegetables. Serve the sliced pork with balsamic-glazed vegetables and quinoa.

Nutrition Facts: Serving Size: 3 Oz. Pork, 1/2 Cup Quinoa & 1 Cup Vegetables
- Exchanges: 3 1/2 Fat, 4 Vegetable, 3 Lean Protein, 1/2 Other Carbohydrate, 1 Starch
- Calories: 490
- Carbohydrates: 44.3g (14% DV)
- Protein: 31g (62% DV)
- Sugars: 14.9g
- Dietary Fiber: 7.9g (32% DV)
- Fat: 21.7g (33% DV)
- Sodium: 653.1mg (26% DV)
- Cholesterol: 73.7mg (25% DV)
- Saturated Fat: 3.5g (18% DV)
- Vitamin A (IU): 10972.2IU (219% DV)
- Folate: 127.3mcg (32% DV)
- Vitamin C: 54.3mg (91% DV)

- Calcium: 88.3mg (9% DV)
- Magnesium: 114.2mg (41% DV)
- Iron: 3.3mg (18% DV)
- Potassium: 1240.4mg (35% DV)
- Thiamin: 0.3mg (25% DV)

DAY FOUR
BREAKFAST

Baked Salmon with Smoky Chickpeas and Greens
This wholesome salmon meal is a great way to incorporate some greens and a zesty
green dressing. Including a weekly dose of dark leafy greens in your diet can help
support brain health. The dish features the Test Kitchen's latest method for chickpea
preparation: seasoning and roasting them to a crispy perfection.

Ingredients:
- 2 tablespoons of extra-virgin olive oil, divided
- 1 ¼ pounds of wild salmon, cut into four portions
- 1 tablespoon of smoked paprika
- 1 can (15 ounces) of no-salt-added chickpeas, rinsed
- 10 cups of chopped kale
- ⅓ cup of buttermilk
- ¼ cup of mayonnaise
- ¼ cup of chopped fresh chives and/or dill, plus extra for garnish
- ¼ teaspoon of garlic powder
- Salt and pepper, divided
- ¼ cup of water

Directions:
1. Preheat the oven to 425 degrees F with racks in the upper and middle thirds.
2. In a medium bowl, mix one tablespoon of oil, smoked paprika, and 1/4
   teaspoon of salt. Toss the chickpeas in this mixture after ensuring they're
   thoroughly dried. Spread them on a rimmed baking sheet and bake on the
   upper rack, stirring them twice during the 30-minute roasting time.
3. Puree the buttermilk, mayonnaise, fresh herbs, 1/4 teaspoon of pepper, and
   garlic powder in a blender until smooth. Set aside.
4. In a large skillet, heat the remaining one tablespoon of oil over medium heat.
   Add the kale and cook for 2 minutes, occasionally stirring. Add water and
   cook until the kale becomes tender, which takes about 5 more minutes.
   Remove from heat and season with a pinch of salt.
5. Remove the chickpeas from the oven and place them on one side of the skillet.
   On the other side, add the salmon portions and season each with the remaining
   1/4 teaspoon of salt and pepper. Bake for 5 to 8 minutes until the salmon is
   just cooked.
6. Drizzle the reserved dressing over the salmon and garnish with additional
   fresh herbs, if desired. Serve with the roasted chickpeas and kale.

Nutrition Facts:
Serving Size: 3/4 Cup Greens, 4 Oz. Salmon, 2 1/2 Tbsp. & 1/4 Cup Chickpeas
Exchanges: 1 Starch, 5 Lean Protein, 1/2 Vegetable, 3 Fat 446.5 calories;
carbohydrates 23.4g 8% DV; protein 37g 74% DV; exchange other carbs 1.5; sugars
2.2g; Fat 21.8g 34% DV; dietary fiber 6.4g 26% DV saturated fat 3.7g 19% DV;
vitamin a iu 5200IU 104% DV; cholesterol 72.9mg 24% DV; vitamin c 51.7mg 86%
DV; calcium 197.8mg 20% DV folate 77.9mcg 20% DV; Iron 3mg 17% DV;
potassium 990.8mg 28% DV; magnesium 99.4mg 36% DV; sodium 556.7mg 22%
DV.

Jackfruit Barbacoa Burrito Bowls

Jackfruit, a tropical fruit with a hearty, meaty texture, serves as a versatile canvas
for this delightful burrito bowl. The jackfruit is cooked in a savory chili sauce,
resulting in a flavorful plant-based alternative to traditional pork or beef.

Ingredients:
- 2 tablespoons olive oil
- 6 garlic cloves, crushed
- 1 cup chopped white onion
- 1 ½ cups unsalted vegetable broth
- 1 medium New Mexico chili, stem and seeds removed
- 1 lime, quartered
- 2 cans (20 ounces each) green jackfruit in brine, rinsed and shredded
- ½ teaspoon kosher salt
- 1 teaspoon chili powder
- ½ teaspoon ground pepper
- 1 cup unsalted canned black beans, rinsed
- 3 cups hot cooked brown rice
- 1 bay leaf
- 2 cups thinly sliced iceberg lettuce
- 1 ⅓ cups chopped plum tomatoes (about 3 medium)
- ½ cup chopped fresh cilantro

Directions:
1. Heat oil over medium-high heat in a medium saucepan. Add garlic, chili, and
   onion. Cook for about 6 minutes, stirring occasionally, until the onion is
   tender and browned. Add broth and bring to a boil. Partially cover and reduce
   heat to medium. Cook for about 10 minutes until the chili is tender. Transfer
   the mixture to a blender. Remove the center blender lid piece to allow steam

to escape, then secure the lid. Place a clean towel over the opening and process for about 45 seconds. Be cautious when blending hot liquids.

2. Return the chili to the pot and add jackfruit, kosher salt, chili powder, bay leaf, and ground pepper. Bring to a simmer over medium-high heat, then cover, and cook for 6 to 8 minutes until slightly thickened. Remove the bay leaf.
3. In each of 4 shallow bowls, place 3/4 cup of rice. Top each serving with a mixture of 1/2 cup lettuce, 3/4 cup jackfruit, 1/3 cup tomatoes, 2 tablespoons cilantro, and 1/4 cup beans. Serve with lime wedges.

Nutrition Facts:

Serving Size: 1 Bowl 450.1 calories; carbohydrates 80.3g 26% DV; protein 9.6g 19% DV; exchange other carbs 5.5; sugars 6.1g; fat 9.4g 14% DV; dietary fiber 22.1g 89% DV saturated fat 1.4g 7% DV; vitamin c 41.3mg 69% DV; vitamin a iu 3019.1IU 60% DV; folate 66.5mcg 17% DV; iron 4.1mg 23% DV; calcium 178.2mg 18% DV; magnesium 109mg 39% DV; sodium 755.5mg 30% DV; potassium 612.5mg 17% DV; thiamin 0.3mg 35% DV.

DAY FIVE

BREAKFAST

Paprika-Roasted Pork Tenderloin with Potatoes and Broccoli

You'd never believe you can create such an elegant dish with just a single baking sheet. While the pork rests, complete this impressive, well-balanced dinner with a simple red pepper sauce (which is equally delightful with chicken). We're confident that this straightforward sheet pan dinner recipe will become a staple in your kitchen.

Ingredients:

- ¾ pound of Yukon Gold potatoes, scrubbed and cut into 1-inch pieces
- 2 cloves of garlic, peeled
- 1 medium red onion, cut into 1-inch pieces
- 2 tablespoons of olive oil, divided
- 2 jarred roasted red bell peppers (6 oz.)
- 1 teaspoon of lemon juice
- 2 tablespoons of low-fat plain Greek yogurt or low-fat sour cream
- 4 cups of broccoli florets (about 1 lb.)
- 1 ½ teaspoons of smoked paprika
- ½ teaspoon of ground pepper, divided
- ¾ teaspoon of salt, divided
- 1 (1-pound) pork tenderloin, trimmed
- 2 teaspoons of Dijon mustard

Directions:
1. Preheat your oven to 425°F and place a large rimmed baking sheet in it.
2. In a medium bowl, combine the potatoes, one clove of garlic, one tablespoon of olive oil, and a quarter teaspoon of salt; toss to coat. Remove the hot baking sheet from the oven and lightly coat it with cooking spray. Spread the potato mixture on the sheet and roast for 15 minutes.
3. While the potatoes are roasting, toss the broccoli with the remaining teaspoon of olive oil, a quarter teaspoon of salt, and a quarter teaspoon of ground pepper in another medium bowl.
4. Place the remaining clove of garlic on a small piece of foil, drizzle it with the remaining teaspoon of oil, and fold the foil into a small packet. In a small bowl, combine the remaining quarter teaspoon of paprika, remaining quarter teaspoon of ground pepper, and remaining quarter teaspoon of salt.
5. Spread the Dijon mustard over the pork tenderloin and coat it with the paprika mixture.
6. Remove the baking sheet from the oven. Move the potatoes and onions to one side and place the pork on the other side. Scatter the seasoned broccoli on the sheet and place the garlic packet where there's space. Roast for about 25 minutes, or until an instant-read thermometer inserted into the thickest part of the pork registers 145°F.
7. While the pork rests, prepare the sauce: carefully unwrap the garlic and transfer it to a mini food processor or blender. Add the roasted red peppers, sour cream (or yogurt), lemon juice, and a quarter teaspoon of ground pepper. Blend until smooth.
8. Slice the pork into 12 pieces. Divide the pork, potatoes, broccoli, and red pepper sauce among four plates. Drizzle the red pepper sauce over the top.

Nutrition Facts:
322.6 calories; carbohydrates 28.7g 9% DV; protein 30g 60% DV; exchange other carbs 2; sugars 5.5g; fat 10.3g 16% DV; dietary fiber 5.3g 21% DV; saturated fat 2.1g 10% DV; cholesterol 76.2mg 25% DV; vitamin A iu 3879.9IU 78% DV; potassium 1246.8mg 35% DV; vitamin C 154mg 257% DV; folate 98.4mcg 25% DV; iron 3.2mg 18% DV; calcium 98.9mg 10% DV; magnesium 83.8mg 30% DV; sodium 730.7mg 29% DV.

Creamy Chicken, Brussels Sprouts, and Mushroom One-Pot Pasta
In this simple one-pot pasta dish, you only need to use a single pot to cook the chicken, vegetables, and noodles. Additionally, by using the same amount of water needed to cook the pasta, you'll retain the starchy goodness that's typically drained with pasta water, yielding a deliciously creamy result.

Ingredients:
- 8 ounces whole-wheat linguine or spaghetti
- 4 cups water
- ¾ teaspoon dried rosemary
- 2 tablespoons chopped fresh chives
- 1 pound boneless, skinless chicken thighs
- 2 cups sliced Brussels sprouts
- 4 cups sliced mushrooms
- 1 ¼ teaspoons dried thyme
- 1 medium onion, chopped
- 4 cloves garlic, thinly sliced
- 2 tablespoons Boursin cheese
- ¾ teaspoon salt

Directions:
1. In a large pot, combine the pasta, chicken, water, Brussels sprouts, onion, garlic, rosemary, thyme, and salt. Bring it to a boil over high heat. Boil, stirring regularly until the pasta is cooked and most of the water has evaporated, which takes about 10 to 12 minutes. Remove from heat and let it sit for 5 minutes, stirring occasionally. Serve with chives sprinkled on top.

Nutritional Information:
Serving: About 1 1/2 Cups Each Exchanges: 1 1/2 Vegetable, 2 1/2 Starch, 2 1/2 Lean Meat 352.5 calories; carbohydrates 41.7g 14% DV; protein 27g 54% DV; exchange other carbs 3; dietary fiber 7.6g 30% DV; saturated fat 3.6g 18% DV; sugars 4.4g; fat 10.3g 16% DV; cholesterol 67.4mg 23% DV; niacin equivalents 8.8mg 68% DV; vitamin A iu 354.8IU 7% DV; vitamin B6 0.4mg 25% DV; folate 68.6mcg 17% DV; vitamin C 27.6mg 46% DV; calcium 63.4mg 6% DV; magnesium 97.3mg 35% DV; iron 3.8mg 21% DV; potassium 567.5mg 16% DV; thiamin 0.3mg 30% DV; sodium 460.9mg 18% DV; percent of calories from protein 29; percent of calories from carbs 45; calories from fat 92.4kcal; percent of calories from fat 25; percent of calories from saturated fat 8.

Family-Style Chicken Spaghetti
(Serves 4, serving size: 2 cups)

Ingredients:
- 2 teaspoons of olive oil
- 8 ounces of uncooked whole-wheat spaghetti

- 2 pints of cherry tomatoes
- 3 garlic cloves, smashed
- 1/4 cup of fresh basil leaves, divided
- 1 medium onion, cut into 1-inch wedges
- 1/2 teaspoon of kosher salt
- 2 tablespoons of unsalted tomato paste
- 8 ounces of shredded skinless, boneless rotisserie chicken breast (about 2 cups)
- 1/2 teaspoon of freshly ground black pepper
- 3 tablespoons of shaved Parmesan cheese

Preparation:

1. Preheat the broiler and line a jelly-roll pan with foil.
2. While the pasta is cooking according to package instructions (omitting salt and fat), combine the oil, garlic, tomatoes, and onion in the prepared pan; toss. Broil for 4-6 minutes. Transfer the mixture from the pan, including any liquid, to a blender. Add two tablespoons of basil and the tomato paste, then securely cover the blender lid. Remove the center of the blender lid and cover with a kitchen towel. Blend until perfectly smooth.
3. Drain the pasta and return it to the pan. Add the tomato sauce, salt, chicken, and pepper. Cook over medium heat until hot. Transfer the spaghetti mixture to a serving platter. Chop the remaining two tablespoons of basil leaves and sprinkle them evenly with Parmesan over the spaghetti.

Nutritional Information:

- Calories: 404
- Saturated Fat: 2.1g
- Total Fat: 7.5g
- Polyunsaturated Fat: 1.1g
- Monounsaturated Fat: 3.3g
- Carbohydrates: 55g
- Protein: 34g
- Cholesterol: 70mg
- Dietary Fiber: 10g
- Sodium: 603mg
- Iron: 3mg
- Sugars: 9g
- Calcium: 137mg
- Estimated Added Sugars: 0g

DAY SIX
BREAKFAST

Family-Style Meatball "Fondue"
Active Time: 30 Minutes
Total Time: 30 Minutes
Servings: 4 (Each serving includes 6 slices of bread, 6 meatballs, and approximately 1/2 cup of sauce)
Ingredients:
- 3/4 cup of chopped zucchini
- Cooking spray
- 1/3 cup of chopped yellow onion
- 12 ounces of ground turkey
- 1/4 teaspoon of kosher salt
- 1/2 teaspoon of dried oregano
- 1 large egg
- 1/4 teaspoon of black pepper
- 8 ounces of sliced cremini mushrooms
- 1 tablespoon of olive oil
- 1 1/2 cups of low-salt marinara sauce
- 2 garlic cloves, minced
- 4 ounces of shredded reduced-fat mozzarella cheese
- 1/4 cup of water
- 24 thin slices from a whole-wheat baguette, toasted

Preparation:
- Step 1: Preheat your oven to 400 degrees F. Line a baking sheet with aluminum foil and cover it with cooking spray.
- Step 2: Place the chopped zucchini between two layers of paper towels and squeeze out the excess moisture. In a bowl, mix the zucchini, ground turkey, chopped onion, dried oregano, kosher salt, black pepper, and the egg. Form this mixture into 24 meatballs, each about one tablespoon in size, and place them on the prepared baking sheet. The turkey mixture may be soft, but it will firm up as the meatballs cook. Bake them at 400°F for approximately 12 minutes or until they are fully cooked.
- Step 3: Meanwhile, heat a large, ovenproof skillet over medium-high heat. Add the olive oil and swirl it around to coat the pan. Add the sliced cremini mushrooms and minced garlic, and cook for about 5 minutes, stirring occasionally, until the mushroom liquid has mostly evaporated. Stir in 1/4 cup of water and the marinara sauce. Reduce the heat to low and simmer for 5

minutes. Return the cooked meatballs to the skillet, leaving any excess liquids behind. Gently swirl them to coat with the sauce. Evenly sprinkle the meatballs with the reduced-fat mozzarella cheese.

- Step 4: Preheat your broiler with the oven rack in the top position. Broil the meatball mixture for about 2 minutes, or until the cheese is melted and bubbly. Serve with toasted baguette slices.

Nutritional Information:
- Calories: 403
- Saturated Fat: 6g
- Total Fat: 21g
- Protein: 31g
- Unsaturated Fat: 12g
- Fiber: 3g
- Carbohydrate: 26g
- Calcium: 26% DV
- Sodium: 693mg
- Sugars: 7g
- Potassium: 15% DV

LUNCH: Sesame-Ginger-Chickpea-Stuffed Sweet Potatoes
Active Time: 40 Minutes
Total Time: 1 Hour 40 Minutes
Servings: 4 (Each serving includes 2 stuffed sweet potato halves)

Ingredients:
- 1 teaspoon of canola oil
- 4 medium sweet potatoes (about 8 oz. each)
- 2 teaspoons of toasted sesame oil
- 1 (15-oz.) can of unsalted chickpeas, rinsed and drained
- 1/2 teaspoon of kosher salt, divided
- 1 teaspoon of garlic powder
- 3 tablespoons of well-stirred tahini
- 1/2 teaspoon of ground ginger
- 1 teaspoon of grated fresh garlic
- 1 teaspoon of grated peeled fresh ginger
- 3 tablespoons of hot water
- 1 teaspoon of rice vinegar
- 2 teaspoons of water
- 4 teaspoons of Sriracha chili sauce

- 1/2 teaspoon each of white and black sesame seeds
- 1/4 cup of thinly sliced green onions

Preparation:
- Step 1: Preheat your oven to 400 degrees F.
- Step 2: Rub the sweet potatoes with canola oil and pierce them liberally with a fork. Bake at 400°F for about 1 hour or until they are tender. Once done, cut the sweet potatoes in half lengthwise and gently score the flesh with the tip of your knife.
- Step 3: Place the well-drained chickpeas on a baking sheet; pat them dry with paper towels. Add the sesame oil and toss the chickpeas. Sprinkle with 1/4 teaspoon of salt, garlic powder, and ground ginger; toss. Bake them at 400°F for about 30 minutes, stirring every 10 minutes.
- Step 4: In a bowl, combine the tahini, fresh garlic, fresh ginger, and rice vinegar. Add three tablespoons of hot water and mix until smooth and slightly runny.
- Step 5: In another bowl, mix the Sriracha sauce with two teaspoons of water. Drizzle about two teaspoons of the tahini mixture over each sweet potato half and sprinkle with the remaining 1/4 teaspoon of salt. Top with the chickpea mixture, more tahini, the Sriracha mixture, green onions, and sesame seeds.

Nutritional Information:
- Calories: 413
- Saturated Fat: 1.3g
- Total Fat: 10.6g
- Polyunsaturated Fat: 4.1g
- Monounsaturated Fat: 4.1g
- Carbohydrate: 69g
- Protein: 12g
- Cholesterol: 0.0mg
- Fiber: 12g
- Sodium: 495mg
- Iron: 3mg
- Sugars: 10g
- Calcium: 136mg
- Estimated Added Sugars: 1g

DINNER: Greek Chopped Salad with Grilled Pita
Active Time: 30 Minutes

Total Time: 30 Minutes
Servings: 4 (Each serving includes about 2 1/4 cups of salad and about 4 pita wedges)

Ingredients:
- 1 large red bell pepper
- Cooking spray
- 2 teaspoons of chopped fresh oregano, divided
- 1/4 cup of olive oil, divided
- 3/8 teaspoon of kosher salt, divided
- 1/2 teaspoon of garlic powder
- 1 tablespoon of white wine vinegar
- 3 (6 1/2-inch) whole-wheat pita rounds
- 2 teaspoons of Dijon mustard
- 1 tablespoon of fresh lemon juice
- 4 cups of chopped romaine lettuce
- 1/4 teaspoon of black pepper
- 1 cup of halved cherry tomatoes
- 2 cups of chopped English cucumber
- 1 (15-oz.) can of unsalted cannellini beans, rinsed and drained
- 2 tablespoons of chopped pitted kalamata olives
- 1 ounce of crumbled feta cheese (about 1/4 cup)

Preparation:
- Step 1: Heat a medium-high grill pan. Cover the pan with cooking spray. Remove the seeds and membranes from the red bell pepper and cut it into pieces. Add the bell pepper to the pan and cook for 4 minutes on each side until it's soft and charred. Remove the bell pepper from the pan and cut it into bite-size pieces.
- Step 2: In a bowl, mix 1 tablespoon of olive oil, 1 teaspoon of chopped fresh oregano, garlic powder, and 1/8 teaspoon of kosher salt. Brush this oil mixture evenly on both sides of all pita rounds. Add the pita rounds to the pan and cook for 2 minutes on each side or until they are well-marked. Slice each pita into six wedges.
- Step 3: In a wide bowl, combine the remaining 3 tablespoons of olive oil, white wine vinegar, lemon juice, and Dijon mustard. Whisk them together. Add the remaining 1 teaspoon of oregano, 1/4 teaspoon of kosher salt, and black pepper. Add the lettuce, charred red bell pepper, cherry tomatoes, cucumber, olives, and beans to the bowl and toss well. Divide the salad into

four servings and top each with an equal amount of crumbled feta cheese. Serve with the grilled pita wedges.

Nutritional Information:
- Calories: 396
- Saturated Fat: 3g
- Total Fat: 19g
- Protein: 12g
- Unsaturated Fat: 12g
- Fiber: 10g
- Carbohydrate: 48g
- Calcium: 12% DV
- Sodium: 684mg
- Sugars: 6g
- Potassium: 21% DV
- Estimated Added Sugars: 0g

DAY SEVEN
BREAKFAST

Tangy Chicken-Farro Bowl
Servings: 4 (Each serving includes 3/4 cup of farro, 3 ounces of chicken, 3 tablespoons of pickles, 1 tablespoon of preserves, and 1 tablespoon of dressing)

Ingredients:
- 2 tablespoons of sugar, split into two portions
- 5 tablespoons of white vinegar, split into five portions
- 1/8 teaspoon of ground allspice
- 5/8 teaspoon of kosher salt, split into two portions
- 2 tablespoons of Dijon mustard
- 2 Persian cucumbers, thinly sliced
- 1 tablespoon of canola oil
- 1/2 teaspoon of dry mustard
- 2 (8.5-ounce) packages of precooked farro
- 2 teaspoons of finely chopped fresh dill
- 1/4 cup of lingonberry preserves
- 2 (6-ounce) rotisserie chicken breasts, skinless and boneless, sliced

Preparation:
- Step 1: In a bowl, combine 1/4 cup of vinegar, 4 teaspoons of sugar, 1/4 teaspoon of salt, and allspice; whisk together. Add cucumbers, toss to coat, and let them stand for 12 minutes. Afterward, drain the cucumbers.
- Step 2: In another bowl, mix Dijon mustard, dry mustard, the remaining one tablespoon of vinegar, the remaining two teaspoons of sugar, and the canola oil. Stir in the water, dill, and 1 1/2 teaspoons of salt.
- Step 3: Prepare the farro according to the package instructions. Divide the cooked farro into four bowls. Arrange the chicken, cucumbers, and farro alongside the preserves. Sprinkle the mustard sauce over the top and add the remaining 3/8 teaspoon of salt.

Nutritional Information:
- Calories: 406
- Saturated Fat: 1.2g
- Total Fat: 7.6g
- Polyunsaturated Fat: 1.6g
- Monounsaturated Fat: 3.3g
- Carbohydrate: 53g

- Protein: 31g
- Estimated Added Sugars: 15g
- Cholesterol: 72mg
- Fiber: 4g
- Sodium: 371mg
- Iron: 3mg
- Sugars: 16g
- Calcium: 44mg

LUNCH: Dilly Salmon Packets with Asparagus

Servings: 4 (Each serving includes 1 fillet and 4 oz. of asparagus)

Ingredients:

- 4 (6-oz.) salmon fillets (approximately 1-inch thick)
- Cooking spray
- 1/4 cup of chopped fresh dill
- 2 tablespoons of unsalted butter
- 1/2 teaspoon of black pepper
- 1/2 teaspoon of kosher salt
- 2 tablespoons of olive oil
- 8 slices of orange
- 1 pound of asparagus, trimmed

Preparation:

- Step 1: Preheat the grill to medium-high heat.
- Step 2: Coat 4 (12-inch-square) pieces of foil with cooking spray. Place one salmon fillet in the center of each piece. Add 1 1/2 teaspoons of butter and 1 tablespoon of dill to each fillet. Sprinkle with salt, pepper, and place orange slices evenly on top. Fold the foil edges over the fillets and seal. Place the packets on the grill, seal side up, cover, and grill for about 12 minutes or until the desired level of doneness is reached. Remove the foil packets from the grill.
- Step 3: Toss the asparagus in a bowl with olive oil. Place the asparagus on the grill and grill for about 5 minutes, turning once, for 3 minutes. Divide the grilled asparagus evenly among four plates. Open the foil packets and top with fillets. Squeeze the orange slices evenly over the fillets.

Nutritional Information:

- Calories: 394
- Saturated Fat: 6.3g

- Total Fat: 23.6g
- Polyunsaturated Fat: 5.3g
- Monounsaturated Fat: 10g
- Carbohydrate: 9g
- Protein: 37g
- Estimated Added Sugars: 0g
- Cholesterol: 109mg
- Fiber: 3g
- Sodium: 319mg
- Iron: 4mg
- Sugars: 5g
- Calcium: 67mg

DINNER: Provolone and Broccoli Rabe Beef Sliders

Total Time: 20 Minutes
Servings: 4 (Each serving includes 2 sliders)

Ingredients:

- 7 ounces of broccoli, trimmed
- Cooking spray
- 1 tablespoon of extra-virgin olive oil
- 1 1/2 tablespoons of red wine vinegar
- 1 pound of 93% lean ground sirloin
- 1 teaspoon of sugar
- 1/2 teaspoon of Worcestershire sauce
- 1 teaspoon of smoked paprika
- 1/4 teaspoon of freshly ground black pepper
- 1/4 teaspoon of kosher salt
- 8 whole-wheat slider buns, each 1-ounce
- 3 slices of reduced-fat provolone cheese, torn into small pieces
- 8 slices of heirloom tomato

Preparation:

- Step 1: Heat a medium-high grill pan. Coat the pan with cooking spray. Add the broccoli and cook for 5 minutes, turning occasionally. Coarsely chop the cooked broccoli. In a small bowl, add the vinegar, oil, and sugar. Add the broccoli and toss.

- Step 2: In a bowl, combine the ground beef, paprika, Worcestershire sauce, salt, and pepper. Form this mixture into eight patties, each about 3 inches wide.
- Step 3: Return the grill pan to medium-high heat, coat it with cooking spray, and add the patties. Cook them for 2 to 3 minutes on one side, then flip and cook for an additional 1 to 2 minutes. Top the patties with the provolone cheese, cover, and cook for another minute, or until the cheese melts.
- Step 4: Place one patty on the bottom half of each bun, add tomato slices, a spoonful of the broccoli mixture, and the top bun halves.

Nutritional Information:
- Calories: 404
- Saturated Fat: 4.8g
- Total Fat: 15.9g
- Polyunsaturated Fat: 2.5g
- Monounsaturated Fat: 6.3g
- Carbohydrate: 32g
- Protein: 38g
- Cholesterol: 71mg
- Fiber: 2g
- Sodium: 573mg
- Iron: 4mg
- Estimated Added Sugars: 6g
- Calcium: 261mg and Sugars: 7g

WEEK TWO MEAL PLAN

DAY ONE
BREAKFAST

Barbeque Chicken with Peach and Feta Slaw
Servings: 4 (Each serving includes 1 1/2 cups of slaw and about 3 1/2 oz. of chicken)

Ingredients:
- 2 tablespoons of sherry vinegar
- 5 tablespoons of olive oil, divided
- 3/8 tsp. of kosher salt, divided
- 1/2 tsp. of freshly ground black pepper, divided
- 1 (12-oz.) package of broccoli slaw
- 2 slices of center-cut bacon, cooked and crumbled
- 1 1/2 cups of sliced fresh peaches
- 1/4 cup of barbecue sauce
- 3 (6-oz.) skinless, boneless chicken breasts, cut crosswise into 1-inch strips
- 1 ounce of crumbled feta cheese (about 1/4 cup)
- 1 tablespoon of chopped fresh chives

Preparation:
Step 1: In a large bowl, whisk together 4 teaspoons of oil, vinegar, 1/4 teaspoon of pepper, and 1/4 teaspoon of salt. Toss the peaches and slaw in the vinegar mixture to coat them gently.
Step 2: Sprinkle the chicken with 1/4 of the remaining teaspoon of pepper and 1/8 of the remaining teaspoon of salt. In a large non-stick skillet, heat the remaining one tablespoon of oil over medium-high heat. Add the chicken to the pan and cook for approximately 6 minutes or until fully cooked. Transfer the chicken to a large bowl and toss it with the barbecue sauce.
Step 3: Divide the slaw mixture equally among 4 plates and top it with the chicken strips. Sprinkle with chives, feta, and bacon.

Nutritional Information:
- Calories: 407
- Fat: 22.5g
- Monounsaturated Fat: 13.7g
- Saturated Fat: 4.4g
- Protein: 33g

- Polyunsaturated Fat: 2.4g
- Fiber: 3g
- Carbohydrate: 16g
- Iron: 2mg
- Cholesterol: 90mg
- Calcium: 67mg
- Sodium: 631mg
- Estimated Added Sugars: 5g
- Sugars: 10g

LUNCH: Mini Veggie Tlayudas
Active Time: 45 Minutes
Total Time: 1 Hour 10 Minutes
Servings: 6 (Each serving is one tlayuda)
Ingredients:
- 2 tablespoons of olive oil
- 1 cup of hulled pumpkin seeds (pepitas)
- 1 minced garlic clove
- 1 teaspoon of ground cumin
- 1/8 teaspoon of freshly ground black pepper
- 1/8 teaspoon of salt
- 1/4 cup of chopped fresh cilantro
- 1 cup of thinly sliced cabbage
- 6 (6-inch) corn tortillas
- 2 tablespoons of fresh lime juice
- 4 ounces of shredded Oaxaca cheese or reduced-fat mozzarella
- 1 1/2 cups of soaked, then fried black beans
- 1 cup of sliced tomatoes
- Cooking spray
- 1 large avocado, thinly sliced

Preparation:
- Step 1: Preheat a low grill.
- Step 2: Heat a small skillet over low heat. Add the pumpkin seeds to the pan and grill for 3 minutes or until lightly browned, stirring often. Transfer the seeds to a spice grinder or mini food processor and process them until a coarse paste forms.
- Step 3: Heat a medium skillet over medium-high heat. Add oil and swirl to coat. Add the ground pumpkin seeds, cumin, and garlic; cook for 3 minutes or until fragrant. Stir in the pepper and salt.

- Step 4: In a medium bowl, combine the cabbage, cilantro, and lime juice, tossing well.
- Step 5: Arrange the tortillas in a single layer on a baking sheet lined with foil. Place the pan on the grill and grill for about 3 minutes until the tortillas begin to crisp.
- Step 6: Divide the pumpkin seed paste equally between the tortillas, spreading it into an even layer. Spoon approximately 1/4 cup of refried beans over each tortilla. Top each tortilla with about 2 1/2 tablespoons of cheese. Place the tortillas coated with cooking spray on the grill rack and grill for 5 minutes or until the cheese melts, and the edges of the tortillas are crisp and browned.
- Step 7: Top with slices of avocado, slaw, and tomato.

Nutritional Information:
- Calories: 390
- Saturated Fat: 5.3g
- Fat: 24.6g
- Polyunsaturated Fat: 6.2g
- Monounsaturated Fat: 11g
- Carbohydrate: 26g
- Protein: 18g
- Cholesterol: 10mg
- Fiber: 9g
- Sodium: 299mg
- Iron: 6mg
- Sugars: 2g
- Calcium: 226mg
- Estimated Added Sugars: 0g

DAY TWO
BREAKFAST

Honey-Ginger Glazed Salmon
Hands-on Time: 30 Minutes
Total Time: 30 Minutes
Serves 4 (Each serving consists of 1 fillet, 1/2 cup rice, and 2 1/4 teaspoons marinade)

Ingredients:
- 1/2 cup honey
- Cooking spray
- 1 1/2-inch piece of finely chopped fresh ginger
- 1/4 cup lower-sodium soy sauce
- 4 (6-ounce) salmon fillets
- 1 grated garlic clove
- 2 cups cooked brown rice

Preparation:
Step 1: Preheat the oven to 400 degrees. Line an aluminum foil jelly-roll pan and lightly brush the foil with cooking spray.
Step 2: In a small saucepan over medium heat, combine the honey and the next three ingredients. Simmer for 2 minutes, stirring frequently. Set aside the marinade at room temperature.
Step 3: Place the salmon fillets in an 8-inch square glass or ceramic baking dish. Pour the cooled marinade over the fillets, turning to coat each one thoroughly. Let it sit for ten minutes.
Step 4: Transfer the fillets to the prepared pan. Strain the marinade into a small saucepan through a sieve, discarding the solids. Over medium heat, bring the marinade to a simmer and cook for 5 minutes. Reserve two tablespoons of marinade in a small bowl, and another three tablespoons in a separate bowl. Discard any remaining marinade.
Step 5: Roast the fillets for 5 minutes at 400 degrees, then remove the pan from the oven.
Step 6: Preheat the broiler to a high setting.
Step 7: Brush the fillets with two tablespoons of reserved marinade and broil on high for 1 to 2 minutes or until the fillets are cooked and glazed. Serve the fillets over the rice and drizzle with the remaining three tablespoons of marinade.

Nutritional Information:
- Calories: 408
- Saturated Fat: 2.2g
- Fat: 10.4g
- Polyunsaturated Fat: 3.6g
- Monounsaturated Fat: 3.5g
- Carbohydrate: 38g
- Protein: 39g
- Cholesterol: 90mg
- Fiber: 2g
- Sodium: 299mg
- Iron: 1mg
- Sugars: 15g
- Calcium: 30mg
- Estimated Added Sugars: 15g

LUNCH: Cherry Tomato Pasta with Prosciutto and Asiago
Hands-on Time: 23 Minutes
Total Time: 23 Minutes
Serves 4 (Each serving size is 1 3/4 cups)

Ingredients:
- 3 tablespoons olive oil, divided
- 8 ounces of uncooked whole-grain penne or rotini
- 1 cup chopped red onion
- 1 ounce thinly sliced prosciutto, coarsely chopped
- 1/8 teaspoon crushed red pepper
- 8 garlic cloves, thinly sliced
- 3 cups multicolored cherry tomatoes, halved
- 1 medium zucchini, quartered lengthwise and sliced
- 2 teaspoons balsamic vinegar
- 1/2 teaspoon kosher salt
- 2 ounces Asiago cheese, grated and divided (about 1/2 cup)
- 1/3 cup chopped fresh flat-leaf parsley

Preparation:
Step 1: Cook the pasta according to the package instructions and drain.
Step 2: Heat 1 tablespoon of oil over medium-high heat in a large skillet. Add the prosciutto and cook until crisp for about 3 minutes. Remove the prosciutto from the pan. Add the remaining two tablespoons of oil to the pan. Add the onion, garlic, and

crushed red pepper and sauté for 4 minutes. Stir in the zucchini and cook for 1 minute. Add the salt and tomatoes and cook for 3 minutes. Stir in the vinegar and pasta and cook for 30 seconds. Remove the pan from the heat and add the parsley and 1 ounce of cheese. Divide the pasta mixture into four bowls and top them with the prosciutto and the remaining 1 ounce of cheese.

Nutritional Information:
- Calories: 405
- Saturated Fat: 4.3g
- Fat: 17.3g
- Polyunsaturated Fat: 2.5g
- Monounsaturated Fat: 9.1g
- Carbohydrate: 53g
- Protein: 15g
- Cholesterol: 17mg
- Fiber: 8g
- Sodium: 499mg
- Iron: 3mg
- Sugars: 11g
- Calcium: 149mg
- Estimated Added Sugars: 0g

DAY THREE
BREAKFAST

Crispy Coconut Chicken Fingers
Preparation Time: 15 Minutes
Cooking Time: 15 Minutes
Serving: 4

Ingredients:
- 1 tsp garlic powder
- 1/2 cup panko breadcrumbs
- 1/2 cup unsweetened shredded coconut
- 2 eggs, beaten
- 1.33 lbs boneless chicken breast (cut into 16 strips)
- Salt and pepper
- 1 tbsp brown sugar

Preparation:
- Step 1: Preheat your oven to approximately 400 degrees. On a large baking sheet, spray with cooking spray.
- Step 2: Season the chicken with salt and pepper. Combine the coconut, panko breadcrumbs, garlic powder, and brown sugar on a tray.
- Step 3: Place the beaten eggs in a shallow bowl next to a plate of breadcrumbs. Dip each chicken strip into the eggs, allowing excess to drip off, and then coat with the coconut breadcrumb mixture. Place each chicken strip on the prepared baking sheet.
- Step 4: Brush the top of the chicken strips with cooking oil. Bake the chicken strips until they turn light brown and their internal temperature reaches 165 degrees, for 7-8 minutes on each side.

Nutrition:
- Calories: 314
- Monounsaturated Fat: 0g
- Protein: 37g
- Total Fat: 11g
- Sodium: 106mg
- Saturated Fat: 7g
- Cholesterol: 167mg
- Total Carbohydrate: 12g
- Polyunsaturated Fat: 0g
- Sugars: 4g

- Dietary Fiber: 2g

LUNCH: Easy Grilled Salmon with Cajun Seasoning
Preparation Time: 15 Minutes
Cooking Time: 15 Minutes
Serving: 4

Ingredients:
- 1/2 tsp garlic powder
- 1 tsp salt
- 1 tsp paprika
- 1/2 tsp onion powder
- 1.33 lbs raw wild salmon
- 1 tbsp olive oil
- 1/2 tsp cumin
- 1 tsp black pepper
- 1/2 tsp oregano
- 1/4 tsp coriander

Preparation:
Step 1: Mix paprika, salt, cumin, black pepper, garlic powder, oregano, coriander, and onion powder together.
Step 2: Rub the salmon with olive oil and apply the spice rub. Let it rest for 15 minutes.
Step 3: Grill over medium-high heat for 8-10 minutes. Adjust the cooking time depending on your grill and salmon's thickness. You can also broil until the fish is cooked through and flakes, for 5-8 minutes.

Nutrition:
- Calories: 257
- Saturated Fat: 3g
- Monounsaturated Fat: 3g
- Total Fat: 13g
- Polyunsaturated Fat: 3g
- Dietary Fiber: 1g
- Sodium: 660mg
- Protein: 33g
- Total Carbohydrate: 1g
- Cholesterol: 68mg
- Sugars: 0g

DINNER: Tilapia Fish Burgers

Preparation Time: 10 Minutes
Cooking Time: 10 Minutes
Serving: 4

Ingredients:
- 1 tsp onion powder
- 1/4 cup Panko breadcrumbs
- 1 lb tilapia
- 1 garlic clove, minced
- 1/2 tsp basil
- 1 egg white
- 1 egg
- 1 tsp salt
- 1/2 tsp black pepper
- 1 tsp paprika
- 4 reduced-calorie hamburger buns
- 1 tomato, sliced
- 1/2 avocado
- 1 tsp vegetable oil
- 2 tbsp Dijon mustard
- 1 cucumber, sliced

Preparation:
- Step 1: Pulse the fish in a food processor until finely chopped.
- Step 2: Combine the breadcrumbs, paprika, egg, mustard, egg white, salt, basil, black pepper, garlic, and onion powder with the fish.
- Step 3: Shape the mixture into patties. If necessary, refrigerate the mixture for 10 minutes before forming patties to help them stay together.
- Step 4: Brush the burgers with vegetable oil.
- Step 5: Cook for approximately 4 minutes on each side in a medium-hot skillet.
- Step 6: Serve on toasted buns with avocado and your preferred burger toppings.

Nutrition:
- Calories: 293
- Monounsaturated Fat: 0g

- Cholesterol: 103mg
- Total Fat: 8g
- Sugars: 4g
- Sodium: 1061mg
- Total Carbohydrate: 28g
- Dietary Fiber: 6g
- Polyunsaturated Fat: 0g
- Protein: 29g
- Saturated Fat: 2g.

DAY FOUR
BREAKFAST

Healthy Korean Ground Beef with Vegetables
Preparation Time: 5 Minutes
Cooking Time: 15 Minutes
Serving: 4

Ingredients:
- 2 tbsp water (more if needed)
- 3 cups mixed Asian vegetables
- 2 garlic cloves, minced
- 2 tbsp. brown sugar (or agave, honey, Stevia to taste)
- 1/4 cup reduced-sodium soy sauce (GF if needed)
- 1 tsp. Asian garlic chili paste (like Sriracha or Sambal Olek)
- 2 tsp sesame oil
- 1 tbsp ginger, minced
- 1.33 lbs. 95% lean ground beef

Preparation:
Step 1: Heat a pan over medium-high heat. Add the Asian vegetables and 2 tbsp of water. Cover and cook for 3-4 minutes or until tender and crisp. Be cautious not to overcook the vegetables. Add a bit more water if the vegetables start to stick or burn. Remove and set aside.
Step 2: In the same pan, add the ground beef. Cook until it's fully cooked, breaking it apart as it cooks.
Step 3: Combine brown sugar, soy sauce, chili paste, sesame oil, garlic, and ginger. Add the mixture to the cooked beef and bring it to a simmer. Cook for an additional 3-4 minutes.
Step 4: Serve the vegetables alongside the beef, drizzling some of the extra sauce on top.

Nutrition:
- Calories: 293
- Monounsaturated Fat: 0g
- Cholesterol: 103mg
- Total Fat: 8g
- Sugars: 4g
- Sodium: 1061mg
- Total Carbohydrate: 28g

- Dietary Fiber: 6g
- Polyunsaturated Fat: 0g
- Protein: 29g
- Saturated Fat: 2g

LUNCH: Grilled Pineapple Barbecue Chicken

Preparation Time: 30 Minutes
Cooking Time: 15 Minutes
Serving: 4

Ingredients:
- 1/2 cup barbecue sauce
- 2 tbsp soy sauce
- 1.33 lbs boneless skinless chicken breast
- 1/4 cup pineapple juice
- 1 garlic clove, minced
- 1 tsp ginger, minced
- 2 cups pineapple, sliced
- 1 tsp Sriracha (optional, more to taste)

Preparation:
Step 1: Mix pineapple juice, barbecue sauce, garlic, soy sauce, ginger, and Sriracha. Marinate the chicken in this mixture for at least 30 minutes or overnight when ready to cook. Allow excess marinade to drip off when removing the chicken.
Step 2: Oil the pineapple slices with cooking oil. Grill the chicken and pineapple for 4-5 minutes on each side or until fully cooked. For thinner chicken, reduce cooking time on each side.
Step 3: In a saucepan, add the remaining marinade. Bring it to a boil and cook for 4-5 minutes until it slightly thickens. Drizzle this over the chicken and pineapple when serving.

Nutrition:
- Calories: 270
- Saturated Fat: 0g
- Monounsaturated Fat: 0g
- Total Fat: 2g
- Sodium: 790mg
- Cholesterol: 74mg
- Protein: 33g
- Polyunsaturated Fat: 0g

- Dietary Fiber: 2g
- Sugars: 19g
- Total Carbohydrate: 25g

DINNER: Sheet Pan Steak Fajitas

Preparation Time: 15 Minutes
Cooking Time: 15 Minutes
Serving: 4

Ingredients:

- 2 limes, juiced
- 3 tbsp fajita seasoning
- 1.33 lbs lean flank steak, sliced thin
- 1 tbsp olive oil
- 2 bell peppers, sliced (any colors)
- 1 red onion, sliced

Preparation:

Step 1: Begin by slicing the flank steak into thin strips using a sharp knife. Depending on the size of the flank steak, you might need to cut longer strips by halving or thirds. Similarly, cut the peppers and onions into small pieces.

Step 2: Toss the beef, bell peppers, and red onion with lime juice, olive oil, and fajita seasoning. Allow it to marinate for 15-30 minutes. You can do this conveniently in a Ziploc bag for easy cleanup when you're short on time.

Step 3: Preheat the oven to 425 degrees. Spray a baking sheet with cooking spray or line it with foil for easier cleanup. Spread out the vegetables and steak in a single layer on the baking sheet.

Step 4: Bake in the oven for 10-12 minutes until the vegetables are tender-crisp and the steak is tender. In the last 2 minutes of cooking, switch the oven to broil to add some char and crispiness to the steak. Please note that when cooked this way, the peppers and onions will still have some bite and texture. If you prefer softer vegetables, put them in the oven for 10 minutes before adding the steak.

Nutrition:

- Calories: 316
- Cholesterol: 104mg
- Total Fat: 13g
- Polyunsaturated Fat: 1g
- Dietary Fiber: 3g
- Monounsaturated Fat: 4g

- Saturated Fat: 5g
- Sugars: 3g
- Total Carbohydrate: 15g
- Sodium: 754mg
- Protein: 34g

DAY FIVE
BREAKFAST

Air Fryer Crispy Chicken Tenders
Preparation Time: 10 Minutes
Cooking Time: 15 Minutes
Serving: 4

Ingredients:
- 1/2 teaspoon seasoned salt
- 1.25 lbs boneless chicken breast tenderloins
- 1/4 cup Panko breadcrumbs
- 2 large eggs, beaten
- 1/2 cup all-purpose flour
- 1/2 cup seasoned breadcrumbs
- 1/2 teaspoon garlic powder
- 1/4 teaspoon black pepper

Preparation:
Step 1: Preheat the air fryer to 375°F. Trim and clean the chicken if needed.
Step 2: Set up your breading station. Place the flour on a plate. On another plate, put the beaten eggs. Then on the third plate, combine seasoned breadcrumbs, garlic powder, Panko breadcrumbs, seasoned salt, and black pepper. Mix this using a fork.
Step 3: Begin by dipping a chicken tender into the flour, allowing the excess to fall off. Then dip it into the egg, letting the excess drip away. Finally, coat the tender thoroughly on all sides with the breadcrumb mixture. Repeat with the remaining tenders.
Step 4: Spray the air fryer rack with cooking spray. Arrange the chicken tenders with some space between them. Cook for 8-10 minutes, or until the tenders are golden brown and cooked through. The exact cooking time may vary depending on their thickness. Make sure all the chicken is fully cooked. Repeat if necessary.

Nutrition:
- Calories: 321
- Monounsaturated Fat: 0g
- Total Carbohydrate: 27g
- Sugars: 1g
- Total Fat: 4g
- Polyunsaturated Fat: 0g
- Dietary Fiber: 1g

- Cholesterol: 93mg
- Saturated Fat: 1g
- Sodium: 398mg
- Protein: 40g

LUNCH: Grilled Chicken Sausages and Vegetables

Preparation Time: 5 Minutes
Cooking Time: 15 Minutes
Serving: 4

Ingredients:
- 1 summer squash, sliced
- 4 chicken sausages (or turkey)
- 2 zucchinis, sliced
- 1/2 cup basil
- 2 tbsp. olive oil
- 2 tomatoes, sliced
- 3 tbsp. balsamic vinegar
- 1 eggplant, sliced
- Salt and pepper

Preparation:
Step 1: Toss the vegetables with olive oil, salt, and pepper.
Step 2: Grill the sausages on a grill until they are fully cooked or heated through. This takes 6-8 minutes per side for raw sausages and 3-4 minutes per side for pre-cooked sausages.
Step 3: Grill the vegetables on the grill or in a grill basket for 3-4 minutes on each side. Chop them coarsely.
Step 4: Add the balsamic vinegar to the vegetables, toss with fresh basil, and season with salt and pepper as needed. Serve the sausages alongside the vegetables.

Nutrition:
- Calories: 285
- Polyunsaturated Fat: 0g
- Total Carbohydrate: 21g
- Saturated Fat: 3g
- Sodium: 503mg
- Total Fat: 13g
- Dietary Fiber: 7g
- Cholesterol: 65mg

- Monounsaturated Fat: 0g
- Sugars: 13g
- Protein: 20g

DINNER: Portobello Burgers with Swiss Cheese and Avocado

Preparation Time: 30 Minutes
Cooking Time: 15 Minutes
Serving: 4

Ingredients:
- 4 slices low-fat Swiss cheese (like Jarlsberg)
- 2 cups arugula
- 1 tbsp olive oil
- 2 tbsp balsamic vinegar
- 1 red onion, sliced
- 1.5 tsp Montreal steak seasoning
- 1 tbsp Worcestershire sauce (vegan if needed)
- 1 tomato, sliced
- 1 tbsp Italian seasoning
- 4 portabella mushroom caps
- 1 avocado, sliced
- 4 reduced-calorie hamburger buns

Preparation:
Step 1: Mix Worcestershire sauce, Italian seasoning, balsamic vinegar, olive oil, and steak seasoning. Marinate the mushrooms in this mixture for at least 30 minutes.
Step 2: When ready to cook, remove the mushrooms from the marinade, letting the excess drip off. Grill them on each side for 4-5 minutes. Just before they are done, add the cheese to allow it to melt. Grill the red onions at the same time. I typically spray them with cooking spray or brush them with olive oil before placing them on the grill.
Step 3: Top the mushrooms with tomatoes, arugula, grilled red onions, and avocado.

Nutrition:
- Calories: 299
- Monounsaturated Fat: 1g
- Total Fat: 13g
- Cholesterol: 10mg
- Dietary Fiber: 9g
- Saturated Fat: 3g

- Total Carbohydrate: 36g
- Sodium: 642mg
- Polyunsaturated Fat: 0g
- Sugars: 9g
- Protein: 15g

DAY SIX
BREAKFAST

Grilled Hawaiian Chicken Sandwiches
Preparation Time: 30 Minutes
Cooking Time: 15 Minutes
Serving: 4

Ingredients:
- ½ tsp Sriracha (optional, more to taste)
- 1/3 cup barbecue sauce
- 1 garlic clove, minced
- 1 jalapeno, sliced
- 1 red onion, sliced
- 1 lb boneless skinless chicken breast
- 3 tbsp pineapple juice
- 1 cup pineapple, sliced
- 4 reduced-calorie hamburger rolls
- 1.5 tbsp soy sauce
- 1 tsp ginger, minced
- 2 cups greens

Preparation:
Step 1: Combine garlic, barbecue sauce, soy sauce, pineapple juice, ginger, and Sriracha. Marinate the chicken in this mixture for at least 30 minutes or overnight.
Step 2: When ready to cook, remove the chicken from the marinade, allowing the excess to drip off. Oil the pineapple slices with cooking oil. Grill the chicken and pineapple on each side for 4-5 minutes or until fully cooked. If the chicken is thinner, reduce the cooking time.
Step 3: Meanwhile, take the leftover marinade and place it in a saucepan. Bring it to a boil and cook until slightly reduced for about 4-5 minutes. Serve it drizzled on the sandwiches.
Step 4: Assemble the sandwiches with sliced red onion, fresh jalapeno, greens, grilled pineapple, and a drizzle of homemade barbecue sauce on the reduced-calorie hamburger rolls.

Nutrition:
- Calories: 287
- Saturated Fat: 0g
- Polyunsaturated Fat: 0g

- Total Fat: 2g
- Cholesterol: 56mg
- Total Carbohydrate: 37g
- Sugars: 15g
- Monounsaturated Fat: 0g
- Dietary Fiber: 4g
- Sodium: 761mg
- Protein: 29g

LUNCH: Healthy Greek Yogurt Pancakes

Preparation Time: 5 Minutes
Cooking Time: 10 Minutes
Serving: 4

Ingredients:
- 2 eggs
- 1 tbsp baking powder
- 1 tbsp maple syrup
- 1 cup skim or unsweetened nut milk
- 1 tsp vanilla extract
- 1.5 cups white whole wheat flour
- 1/2 cup nonfat plain Greek yogurt (or flavored)

Preparation:
Step 1: In a bowl, whisk together milk, eggs, yogurt, vanilla extract, and maple syrup.
Step 2: Add baking powder and flour. Stir until just combined; avoid over-mixing.
Step 3: Preheat a nonstick griddle or skillet over medium heat. Grease with cooking spray. Pour approximately 1/4 cup of batter per pancake. Cook for 3-4 minutes until bubbles form and start to pop. Flip and cook until cooked through.

Nutrition:
- Calories: 262
- Total Fat: 3g
- Cholesterol: 94mg
- Saturated Fat: 1g
- Polyunsaturated Fat: 0g
- Dietary Fiber: 1g
- Monounsaturated Fat: 0g
- Sodium: 348mg

- Sugars: 8g
- Total Carbohydrate: 45g
- Protein: 13g

DINNER: Sheet Pan Chicken Fajitas
Preparation Time: 30 Minutes
Cooking Time: 15 Minutes
Serving: 4

Ingredients:
- 1 tbsp olive oil
- 1 red onion, sliced
- 1.33 lbs boneless chicken breasts, sliced thin
- 2 limes, juiced
- 3 tbsp fajita seasoning
- 2 bell peppers, sliced (any colors)

Preparation:
Step 1: Toss chicken, red onion, and bell peppers with olive oil, lime juice, and fajita seasoning. Let them marinate for 30 minutes. You can use a Ziploc bag for this for easier cleanup.

Step 2: Preheat the oven to 400 degrees. Spray a baking sheet with cooking spray or line it with foil for easier cleaning.

Step 3: Arrange the chicken and vegetables in a single layer on the baking sheet. Place it in the oven and cook until the chicken is nearly cooked through and the vegetables are tender-crisp, for about 10-12 minutes. For the last 2 minutes of cooking, broil to add some crispiness and char to the chicken. Note that the onions and peppers will retain some bite and texture when cooked this way. If you prefer softer vegetables, put them in the oven for 10 minutes before adding the chicken.

Nutrition:
- Calories: 257
- Monounsaturated Fat: 0g
- Saturated Fat: 1g
- Total Carbohydrate: 15g
- Total Fat: 5g
- Sugars: 3g
- Sodium: 722mg
- Cholesterol: 74mg
- Dietary Fiber: 3g
- Polyunsaturated Fat: 0g and Protein: 33g

DAY SEVEN
BREAKFAST

Grilled Lemon Chicken with Tzatziki
Preparation Time: 3 Hours
Cooking Time: 15 Minutes
Serving: 4

Ingredients:
- 1 minced garlic clove
- Juice and zest of half a lemon
- 1.33 lbs of boneless, skinless chicken breast
- 2 tsp of dried oregano
- 2 tbsp of extra virgin olive oil
- 0.5 tsp of dried thyme
- 1 tbsp of chopped dill
- 3 minced garlic cloves (or garlic powder)
- 0.5 cup of plain low-fat yogurt
- Salt and pepper
- 0.5 English cucumber (or Persian cucumbers)

Preparation:
Step 1: Begin by preparing the chicken breasts. To create smaller pieces from larger ones, cut the chicken in half. Then, evenly pound the chicken to ensure uniform thickness, especially in thicker areas.
Step 2: Whisk together lemon juice, olive oil, lemon zest, oregano, garlic, salt, thyme, and pepper. Place the chicken in a Ziploc bag or container and marinate in the refrigerator for a minimum of 2 hours, or up to 6 hours. Rotate the chicken a few times during marination to ensure an even coat.
Step 3: Prepare tzatziki by grating the cucumber and removing excess moisture using a paper towel or cheesecloth. Combine it with lemon zest, lemon juice, salt, dill, and pepper into the yogurt. Refrigerate for at least 1 hour.
Step 4: When you're ready to cook, preheat the grill. Remove the chicken from the marinade and allow excess marinade to drip off. Grill each side for 4-6 minutes, or until it reaches a temperature of 160-165 degrees. Allow the chicken to rest for 5 minutes before serving.

Nutrition:
- Calories: 261
- Monounsaturated Fat: 0g

- Total Fat: 9g
- Sodium: 78mg
- Saturated Fat: 1g
- Dietary Fiber: 2g
- Polyunsaturated Fat: 0g
- Sugars: 3g
- Total Carbohydrate: 6g
- Cholesterol: 76mg
- Protein: 35g

LUNCH: Roasted Italian Sausages with Potatoes, Peppers, and Onions

Preparation Time: 30 Minutes
Cooking Time: 10 Minutes
Serving: 4

Ingredients:
- 1 green pepper
- 0.5 tsp red pepper flakes
- 4 lean turkey Italian sausages
- 1 chopped onion
- 1.33 lbs red potatoes, washed and chopped (Sweet potatoes can be used as a Paleo substitute)
- 1 tbsp Italian seasoning
- 2 red peppers
- 4 minced garlic cloves
- 0.25 cup low-sodium chicken broth

Preparation:
Step 1: Preheat the oven to 400 degrees.
Step 2: In a glass baking dish, combine the onion, potatoes, garlic, and peppers. Sprinkle the red pepper flakes, salt, olive oil, pepper, and Italian seasonings with the chicken broth. Use your hands and a spoon to mix them together. Pierce the sausages with a fork and nestle them among the vegetables.
Step 3: Bake for 30-35 minutes until the vegetables are cooked and tender. If the vegetables don't brown, place them under the broiler for 3-4 minutes.

Nutrition:
- Calories: 314
- Monounsaturated Fat: 0g
- Saturated Fat: 3g

- Total Fat: 11g
- Cholesterol: 60mg
- Polyunsaturated Fat: 0g
- Total Carbohydrate: 35g
- Dietary Fiber: 5g
- Sugars: 7g
- Sodium: 707mg
- Protein: 21g

DINNER: Baked Carrot Cake Oatmeal with Cream Cheese Glaze

Preparation Time: 10 Minutes
Cooking Time: 45 Minutes
Serving: 6

Ingredients:
- 0.25 tsp allspice
- 0.25 tsp ground ginger
- 2 cups rolled oats
- 1 tsp cinnamon
- 0.5 cup natural applesauce or pineapple
- 0.25 cup reduced-fat cream cheese
- 2 tbsp unsweetened shredded coconut
- 0.25 cup raisins
- 0.25 cup maple syrup (adjust to taste)
- 1 cup chopped fresh carrots
- 0.5 tsp vanilla extract
- A pinch of salt
- 2 cups unsweetened almond milk
- 2 eggs
- 1 tbsp chia seeds (optional)
- 1 tbsp powdered sugar (or maple syrup)
- 0.125 tsp nutmeg (optional)
- 1 tbsp warm water

Preparation:
Step 1: Preheat the oven to 400°F. Grease an 8x8 baking dish with cooking spray.
Step 2: In a bowl, mix oats, applesauce, carrots, coconut, raisins, spices, chia seeds, and salt. You can add walnuts or pecans for a more traditional carrot cake flavor.
Step 3: In another bowl, whisk together almond milk, maple syrup, eggs, and vanilla extract. Combine this mixture with the oatmeal mixture.

Step 4: Pour the mixture into the baking dish and bake until the oatmeal is fully set and lightly browned, about 40-50 minutes.

Step 5: Meanwhile, make the glaze by beating together powdered sugar, milk, cream cheese, and vanilla. You can microwave the cream cheese briefly to make it easier to stir.

Step 6: Once the baked oatmeal is ready, let it cool for 15 minutes or more. Drizzle the glaze on top and serve. Leftovers can be stored in the fridge for 4-5 days.

These paraphrased versions provide a clear and concise understanding of the recipes while preserving the key details.

CHAPTER 3
Crafting Your Anti-Inflammatory Diet

Our bodies may be internally aflame, and some of our habits act as fuel for this fire. How can we extinguish or at least manage this blaze? To simplify, inflammation is the body's chemical response aimed at defending itself. Its purpose is to eliminate harmful elements like bacteria, damaged cells, and irritants, marking the initial step toward healing. Inflammation triggers an immune system response. Initially, inflammation is beneficial as it serves for protection. However, excessive or chronic inflammation can lead to serious health issues. Inflammation manifests through five key symptoms: pain, heat, redness, swelling, and impaired function.

The primary causes of inflammation include chronic inflammation, dietary choices, exposure to environmental toxins (in water, food, and air), physiological stress, intensive exercise or endurance activities, emotional trauma, age, and autoimmune conditions. Every food we consume elicits a response from our bodies. Many modern diets include foods that exacerbate inflammation, such as fried foods, processed items, refined foods, excess coffee, alcohol, and carbohydrates.

An anti-inflammatory diet primarily features natural, nutrient-rich foods, devoid of processed items and emphasizing organic and safe options. Key components of this diet include battling inflammation with healthy fats, especially those rich in Omega-3 fatty acids. Fatty fish like sardines, tuna, herring, and anchovies, along with extra virgin coconut oil, olive oil, avocado oil, and walnuts are all beneficial. Rich antioxidant-rich fruits and vegetables include onions, lettuce, sweet potatoes, garlic, broccoli, and leafy greens, alongside blueberries, papaya, strawberries, and bananas. High-quality protein, preferably organic, grass-fed meats and eggs, plays a crucial role. Herbs like ginger, curcumin, turmeric, oregano, and rosemary also contain ingredients that reduce inflammation and inhibit harmful free radical development.

However, some foods must be avoided at all costs on an anti-inflammatory diet. These pro-inflammatory foods include processed foods, fast food (especially deep-fried items), omega-6 fats commonly found in oils like sunflower and soy oil, wheat-based and gluten-containing products, trans fats, sugar-laden meals, bacon, and margarine.

To embark on an anti-inflammatory diet, begin by eliminating pro-inflammatory foods. Even if you're not currently dealing with inflammation, adopting this diet can enhance your overall health and support weight loss. The next step involves incorporating anti-inflammatory foods into your diet, starting with healthy omega-3 fats and cooking with extra virgin olive oil or coconut oil. Replace snacks like chips with nuts and opt for fresh fish or high-quality fish oil supplements. If you don't already consume plenty of fruits and vegetables, now is the time to introduce them into your diet. The variety they offer in flavors and nutritional benefits is a key advantage.

Consider drinking green tea, as it is well-documented to be anti-inflammatory, thanks to its flavonoids. Experiment with herbs and spices in your cooking to replace more commonplace flavor enhancers like salt, sugar, and mayonnaise. Additionally, it's essential to identify and eliminate problematic foods from your diet, especially if you notice intolerance or adverse reactions. For example, wheat and gluten-containing foods are known to cause issues for some individuals. Gradually eliminate suspected culprits one by one to pinpoint the source of your problems."

Addressing Inflammation with Anti-Inflammatory Foods

Are there specific dietary regimens designed to alleviate inflammation, and do they indeed yield positive outcomes? Research has established a connection between our dietary choices and the inflammatory processes occurring within our bodies. Notably, certain food constituents have been identified as capable of mitigating inflammation, while others have the potential to exacerbate it. Nevertheless, there remain numerous intricacies surrounding the intricate interplay of diet and inflammation, and as of now, there is insufficient scientific evidence to delineate which specific foods or food categories might be particularly advantageous for individuals afflicted by arthritis. However, a growing clarity is emerging regarding how best to structure one's diet to curtail inflammation.

So, why is the matter of inflammation of such paramount concern? Inflammation serves as the body's inherent defense mechanism against illnesses and injuries. When an aberration occurs, the immune system orchestrates inflammation to either obliterate the intruder or facilitate the healing of an injury. Inflammation typically manifests as swelling, discomfort, increased temperature, and visible redness, and it tends to subside as the underlying issue is resolved, indicative of a salubrious process.

Notably, chronic inflammation represents an enduring form of inflammation, a state familiar to individuals suffering from rheumatoid arthritis, lupus, psoriasis, and other disorders classified under the "inflammatory" arthritis category. Chronic inflammation is an entity that refuses to abate; the aforementioned types of arthritis, which encompass autoimmune components, serve as perpetrators that impel unrelenting inflammation, devoid of the natural mechanisms to cease this inflammatory response. Unmitigated inflammation, coupled with consequential damage to tissues and the potential for lifelong disability, may precipitate a myriad of other medical complications.

Compelling evidence has revealed inflammation's propensity to foster atherosclerosis, a condition associated with an augmented risk of heart disease attributed to the accumulation of fatty deposits along arterial linings. Furthermore, elevated levels of inflammatory proteins have been documented in the bloodstream of individuals with cardiovascular conditions. The ramifications of inflammation extend beyond cardiovascular ailments, encompassing obesity, asthma, diabetes, Alzheimer's disease, and even cancer. It is the consensus among scientists that persistent, albeit subtle, inflammation in the body can provoke an array of adverse consequences. Substantive research posits that dietary choices bear the potential to ameliorate inflammation, suggesting that an anti-inflammatory diet might exert a positive influence on various health conditions.

In the quest to identify foods conducive to inflammation reduction, researchers have delved into the dietary habits of our forebears, positing that these dietary practices align more harmoniously with the body's inherent capacity to metabolize and harness nutrients from the foods and beverages we ingest. The diet of our distant ancestors predominantly featured wild game meats such as venison and boar, alongside an assortment of wild vegetables comprising leafy greens, fruits, and berries. The epoch preceding the advent of agriculture, dating back approximately 10,000 years, was bereft of cereal grains and had a paucity of dairy and processed or refined foods. The contemporary diet markedly contrasts this primitive culinary landscape, characterized by its high consumption of meats, both lean and saturated (or deficient) fats, processed foods, and minimal physical activity. Furthermore, the ubiquity of modern food availability at the click of a mouse on our computers underscores the substantial departure of current lifestyles and dietary patterns from the physiological framework of our bodies. Our genetic makeup has undergone negligible changes since antiquity, making it incommensurate with the drastic alterations to our diets and behaviors over the past half-century to a century. This incongruity between our diet and our genetic heritage, along with the substantial surge in the consumption of certain foods, particularly inordinate quantities of specific types, has engendered deleterious health consequences.

Within our foods, two notable nutrients have prevailed for millennia: omega-3 and omega-6 fatty acids, components vital for standard growth and development as they are integral to virtually all cell types. Notably, both omega-3 and omega-6 fatty acids play pivotal roles in mediating inflammatory responses. Several studies have elucidated the potency of specific sources of omega-3 fatty acids in reducing inflammation, while omega-6 sources have been incriminated for their propensity to exacerbate inflammatory processes. At present, the prevailing predicament is that the typical American diet manifests an approximate omega-6 to omega-3 ratio that is fifteen-fold higher than historical consumption. The dietary patterns of our remote ancestors were characterized by a harmonious equilibrium in the intake of omega-3 and omega-6 fatty acids, which ostensibly facilitated regulatory control over inflammatory responses. The present disparity in omega-3 and omega-6 consumption in our diets is postulated to underlie the escalating prevalence of inflammation within our bodies.

So, why has the consumption of omega-6 fatty acids proliferated so extensively? Omega-6 fatty acids are prevalent in vegetable oils, including safflower, corn, cottonseed, sunflower, and soy oils, along with derivatives such as margarine. Furthermore, many of the processed snack products available today are inundated with these vegetable oils, having replaced conventional sources of fats, such as butter and lard, based on the prevailing nutritional knowledge of the era. The repercussions of adhering to this counsel have arguably led to an augmented intake of omega-6 fatty acids, thus fostering an imbalance between omega-6 and omega-3 fatty acid levels within the modern diet.

Omega-6 fatty acids can also be traced to several common foods, including meats and egg yolks. Notably, grain-fed animals, such as cattle, sheep, pigs, and poultry, epitomize examples of meat products replete with omega-6 fatty acids. In the United States, a substantial proportion of meat derives from grain-fed livestock, as distinct from their counterparts, which feature fewer fatty acids. By contrast, wild game meats such as venison and certain seafood varieties, such as squid, stand as exceptions characterized by higher levels of omega-3 fatty acids and reduced levels of omega-6. It is essential to underscore that both animal and plant-based foods encompass omega-3 constituents. Importantly, our bodies demonstrate a greater capacity to metabolize animal-derived omega-3 fatty acids into anti-inflammatory compounds in comparison to their plant-derived counterparts. Furthermore, plant-based foods harbor a multitude of safe compounds, a considerable proportion of which possess anti-inflammatory properties, hence warranting their collective retention within our diets.

Incorporating a profusion of omega-3 fatty acids into our diets can be achieved through the consumption of fatty fish, especially those sourced from cold waters. While salmon enjoys widespread recognition for its omega-3 content, it is imperative to acknowledge the comparable omega-3 abundance in mackerel, anchovies, herring, striped bass, and bluefish. In addition to the type of fish, the source of the seafood is of import, as wild-caught fish is generally deemed to represent a superior reservoir of omega-3 fatty acids relative to farm-raised counterparts.

Additionally, omega-3 enriched eggs constitute a viable dietary choice. A profusion of plant-based sources of omega-3 fatty acids can be located within an assortment of leafy greens like kale, spinach, and chard, as well as flaxseed, wheat germ, walnuts, and their respective oils. It is also feasible to procure omega-3 fatty acids, often in the form of fish oil, through dietary supplements, with certain instances showcasing the potential to deliver therapeutic benefits. Nevertheless, it is incumbent upon individuals to consult with healthcare professionals before initiating omega-3 supplementation, particularly when using prescription omega-3 supplements, in light of concerns pertaining to the purity and quality of over-the-counter offerings available at health food stores and supermarkets.

Concomitant with efforts to enhance the intake of anti-inflammatory omega-3 fatty acids, individuals must remain cognizant of the fat content and composition of the foods they consume. The rejection of pro-inflammatory fats, characterized as saturated fats within meats and high-fat dairy products, along with the concomitant prioritization of anti-inflammatory fats, represents a crucial dietary modality for managing inflammation and safeguarding health."

Trans-fats, while relatively recent entrants in the realm of cardiovascular ailments, have established a presence, lurking within packaged consumables and snacks, their presence betraying them through diligent label perusal. Often manifesting as partially hydrogenated oils, most frequently soy and cottonseed oils, these covert trans-fats are not limited to industrially engineered substances but can also appear in trace amounts within animal-derived comestibles.

The prevailing notion is that trans-fats contribute to the pro-inflammatory proclivity of our bodily systems, and the volumes we currently ingest have skyrocketed to unprecedented levels.
Antioxidants, the stalwart compounds thwarting the usurpation of our physiological domains by free radicals generated during inflammatory processes, are prevalent in bounteous proportions within plant-based sustenance. Inhabitants of this verdant kingdom include vegetables, berries, seeds, and nuts, and they are teeming with these protective antioxidants. The reign of antioxidant-richness extends to the domain of culinary oils, with olive oil and walnut oil standing as formidable sources of these potent compounds. These nutritionally vital constituents are often marked by vibrant pigments and are the cornerstones of healthful sustenance. They grace the spectrum of colors present in fruits and vegetables, from the verdant leafy greens to the low-starch stalwarts like broccoli and cauliflower, all the way to the vibrant allure of berries, tomatoes, and the flamboyant orange and yellow hues characterizing various fruits and vegetables.

Arthritis has piqued the curiosity of inquisitive minds, sparking numerous investigations into the nexus between dietary choices and this ailment, particularly rheumatoid arthritis (RA). Researchers have traversed the terrain of dietary inquiries, embarking on extensive explorations of diverse diets and their impact on RA. An intriguing revelation emerges from these studies, with a compendium of research suggesting that diets rich in omega-3 fatty acids exert a discernible influence on ameliorating RA symptoms. Additional insights have unearthed the efficacy of diets balancing omega-3 and omega-6 fatty acids at a ratio of 2 to 3, a stark divergence from the typical dietary ratios, which often extend to an alarming 15 to 1. This pivotal dietary shift towards equilibrium, as opposed to the existing disproportionate status quo, wields the potential to mitigate inflammation among RA-afflicted individuals. Furthermore, explorations into omega-3 consumption have yielded promising results, indicating a diminished need for non-steroidal anti-inflammatory drugs (NSAIDs), like naproxen and ibuprofen (commonly known as Advil and Motrin), when incorporating omega-3 into the dietary regimen.

However, it is imperative to underscore that the body of research, while promising, remains insufficient to unequivocally affirm the tangible benefits of a specific anti-inflammatory diet for assuaging arthritis symptoms. This caveat should not be misconstrued as a condemnation of dietary interventions; rather, it underscores the nascent stage of scientific understanding and leaves the door ajar for potential future revelations. Consequently, diet, when harmoniously conjoined with exercise and medicinal approaches, may emerge as one among several modalities to alleviate the effects of arthritis in the days to come.

The recourse need not be a complete regression to a Neolithic era subsistence, akin to our primitive forebears inhabiting caves. A judicious and contemporary approach lies in consummate alignment with the dietary recommendations of the present. A primary strategy in this quest encompasses the harmonization of current dietary staples with nutrient-rich victuals that resonate with the historical backdrop of anti-inflammatory nourishment. The prescription is simple: supplant omega-6-rich provisions with omega-3-abundant fare, reduce the frequency of meat and poultry ingestion while augmenting the consumption of fatty fish, and integrate an assortment of vibrant fruits and vegetables. In a striking departure from our ancestral dietary patterns, whole grains, albeit absent in our antiquity, merit inclusion due to their wealth of essential nutrients and anti-inflammatory compounds, as long as they retain their unprocessed essence. It is paramount to recognize that an overindulgence in high-sugar and refined white flour products is a recipe for fomenting inflammation, accentuating the importance of moderation in this context.

The knowledge underpinning our comprehension of human physiology and dietary influences bolsters the age-old adage "You are what you eat." However, our understanding is a work in progress, and comprehensive validation of the tangible benefits of an anti-inflammatory diet is contingent on our genetic disposition and the state of our well-being. Unfortunately, equivocations persist on this front, leaving the verdict still pending. It is pivotal to acknowledge that dietary considerations represent just one facet of a multifaceted narrative. The dimensions of physical activity are undeniable, with sedentary proclivities in stark contrast to our forebears, who led physically engaging lives. Furthermore, the disparity in body composition, with our modern profiles characterized by excess adiposity, emerges as another facet of the narrative. Importantly, adipose tissue itself constitutes a dynamic entity capable of producing inflammatory compounds.

The selection of anti-inflammatory foods adheres to a principle where nutritional choices align with the physiological requisites of the body. The path to dietary health is not necessarily a regression to the rudimentary diets of our forebears; rather, it calls for the adoption of a balanced diet that harmoniously accommodates the nutritional proclivities rooted in antiquity. An enlightened dietary approach necessitates a recalibration, one that elevates the prominence of omega-3-rich foods while constricting the realm of omega-6 dominance. It also advocates for moderation in the consumption of meat and poultry, supplemented by the incorporation of oily fish and an array of colorful fruits and vegetables. Although whole grains did not form part of our ancestral dietary heritage, they now constitute a valuable addition, provided they remain unprocessed, preserving their complement of beneficial nutrients and anti-inflammatory agents. A careful evaluation of sugar-laden and white flour-laden dietary elements is prudent, as these can inadvertently incite inflammatory processes. These dietary insights illuminate the intrinsic connection between what we consume and our bodily well-being, ushering in an era where the maxim "You are what you eat" carries newfound significance. Nonetheless, the full exposition of the benefits encapsulated within the realm of anti-inflammatory diets remains an evolving narrative, inexorably influenced by our genetic endowment and the evolving landscape of health.

Anti-Inflammatory Foods which can be incorporated for Pain Relief

Although an increasing number of Americans are turning to conventional homeopathic and natural remedies to address ailments such as arthritis, gout, and assorted muscle and joint discomforts, the simplest and most cost-effective approach to home remedies involves incorporating certain key foods into the American diet. A curated list of these healthful, anti-inflammatory food items is readily available for consideration.

At the pinnacle of this list are fish, renowned for their bounteous reservoirs of anti-inflammatory omega-3 fatty acids, with a particular emphasis on cold-water denizens such as salmon, tuna, and mackerel. The prevailing scientific consensus underscores the efficacy of introducing fish or fish oil into one's dietary regimen for the express purpose of mitigating inflammation. However, the discerning consumer is encouraged to exercise due diligence in their fish selection, as the choice between wild and farmed fish is a matter of considerable debate. Wild fish, by virtue of their natural diets and exercise routines, tend to outshine their farmed counterparts in terms of nutrient density and reduced fat content.

This discrepancy manifests as an approximate 20% disparity, with farmed fish harboring higher fat content and diminished protein levels. Notably, the sources of omega-3 essential fatty acids, such as small fish, shrimp, and red krill, consume wild fish, thus serving as the origin of the surplus of omega-3 EFAs in these marine ecosystems. In contrast, farmed fish subsist on fishmeal pellets primarily derived from ground fish like mackerel, sardines, anchovies, and various smaller species, which, regrettably, lack high concentrations of omega-3 EFAs as compared to their wild counterparts. It is pertinent to acknowledge that farmed fish often undergo a process of color enhancement in their diets to replicate the vivid red hues characteristic of their wild counterparts, particularly in the case of salmon.

Further complexities arise as farmed fish find themselves confined within overcrowded net enclosures or cages, leading to a reliance on antibiotics to manage infections, diseases, and parasites. This compels an informed consumer to exercise caution when confronted with the issue of high mercury levels, a concern that extends to both wild and farmed fish. In wild fish, elevated mercury levels are linked to pollution in their native waters, while farmed fish face mercury contamination through their dietary intake. To mitigate these risks, it is advisable to abstain from consuming fish skin, where mercury tends to accumulate in significant quantities.

Turning the spotlight to extra virgin olive oil, this culinary gem emerges as a veritable font of oleic acid, an anti-inflammatory marvel. Moreover, olive oil stimulates insulin function, thereby facilitating the reduction of blood sugar levels. While it may not be the ideal choice for deep-frying endeavors due to its relatively low smoke point, it remains an excellent option for health-conscious cooking methods such as sautéing and braising. In the realm of dietary oils, the discerning consumer is advised to opt for olive oil or trans-fat-free shortenings, as these alternatives transcend their less healthful counterparts.

Another addition to the anti-inflammatory roster comprises nuts rich in oleic acid, including the likes of cashews and walnuts. These kernel-rich edibles also offer an array of healthful constituents, including fiber, omega-3 fatty acids, protein, and various phytochemicals. However, moderation is the watchword for nut consumption, as some varieties harbor a noteworthy fat content.

On this gastronomic journey towards mitigating inflammation, grapes constitute a noteworthy inclusion, particularly those endowed with elevated levels of flavonoids. These compounds are touted for their anti-inflammatory attributes, as evidenced by research conducted at the Johns Hopkins University School of Medicine. This study yielded compelling evidence of the pain and inflammation-reducing properties of powdered grapes, especially when applied to a rat model of arthritis, in which the rodents exhibited knee inflammation induced by chemical injections.

Cherries, especially the tart variants, represent an abundant source of antioxidants, boasting significant quantities of anthocyanins, among the most potent antioxidants known to science. These anthocyanins are responsible for the rich red hues that grace the cherry's exterior. Additionally, research conducted by scientists and colleagues affiliated with the Agricultural Research Service (ARS) posits that cherries may not only alleviate the painful symptoms of arthritis but also reduce the risk of other inflammatory conditions, such as cardiovascular disease and cancer.

A remarkable staple in the sphere of anti-inflammatory victuals is green tea, characterized by the presence of flavonoids known as "catechins." This tea, distinguished by its unfermented nature, retains an impressive catechin content, a feature that sets it apart from other teas subjected to the processing and fermentation stages. When compared to its counterparts, green tea exhibits a significant advantage, with an approximate 27% catechin content, dwarfing oolong (partially fermented) tea at 23% and black tea (fully fermented) at approximately 4%. Animal-based experiments underscore the substantial influence of green tea in curtailing the incidence of arthritis, as it orchestrates changes within the immune system as it combats this ailment. Nonetheless, it is important to note that, as with any dietary element, individuals may develop allergies, with some experiencing headaches after consuming tea. This calls for a vigilant awareness of one's own bodily responses and a willingness to heed the feedback provided by one's constitution.

Leafy greens, in the form of green, leafy vegetables such as spinach and kale, make a noteworthy addition to the arsenal of anti-inflammatory foods. These verdant delights are packed with essential constituents such as fiber, antioxidants, and omega-3 fatty acids. For the health-conscious consumer, it is prudent to explore the organic produce aisle or exercise thorough washing of non-organic items to remove pesticides and chemicals, which tend to accumulate on the leaves.

The formidable broccoli, in the company of its cruciferous cousins like cauliflower, yields a compound known as 3,3'-diindolylmethane (DIM), celebrated for its inflammation-fighting prowess and immune-boosting capabilities. These super-vegetables also harbor a wealth of sulfur, a phytonutrient that augments liver function, enhancing the body's innate detoxification capabilities. It is crucial to underscore the significance of preserving the beneficial nutrients present in these vegetables by opting for raw consumption or cooking methods that do not undermine their nutritional value. This stands in contrast to certain cooking techniques, such as boiling or frying, which can deplete the nutrient content of various vegetables, particularly when the freezing process is employed.

Inclusion of apples and red onions in the anti-inflammatory dietary regimen is justified by the presence of quercetin, a chemical compound endowed with anti-inflammatory properties, alongside other potent antioxidants. Notably, the majority of quercetin is concentrated in the skin of these fruits, emphasizing the importance of not peeling apples before consumption, as the skin is the very source of their rich red hue. This advice extends to all fresh fruits and vegetables, as an extensive rinsing process is advisable to remove traces of pesticides and fertilizers, which tend to cling to their exteriors.

Finally, the essential role of water, our life-sustaining elixir, merits recognition in the context of anti-inflammatory dietary strategies. Consuming fresh, clean water remains a cornerstone of healthful living, with over 70% of the human body being composed of water. A consistent influx of this precious resource plays a pivotal role in the efficient flushing of contaminants from various bodily systems, including muscles, joints, and the circulatory network. Given the proliferation of bottled water in recent years, a spirited debate has arisen regarding the relative merits of tap water versus bottled water.

The discerning consumer is encouraged to undertake an exploration of the differences and make an informed choice. A plethora of bottled water options now graces the market, spanning spring water, mineral water, and sparkling water. Some of these offerings derive from natural, uncontaminated sources, while more than

25% of bottled water originates from municipal water sources. The pursuit of a hydrated existence is incumbent upon each individual, and the choice between tap water and bottled water must align with personal preferences and priorities.

Simple Adjustments for Improved Health

Numerous trendy diets promise rapid transformations in appearance and well-being. The market inundates consumers with products claiming to enhance skin health and smoothness. In a society that places great emphasis on looking good and staying healthy, there exists a diet that can genuinely promote well-being and extend one's lifespan.

The anti-inflammatory diet offers multifaceted benefits, which makes it surprising that more individuals have not adopted this comfortable lifestyle change. Neither have health and beauty experts fully embraced this novel approach to weight loss, appearance enhancement, and anti-aging. In reality, the anti-inflammatory diet has the potential to deliver on what many diets promise while also promoting longevity.

To embark on the anti-inflammatory diet journey, start by keeping a weekly food journal. During this initial week, adhere to your regular eating habits without any modifications. Once the week is over, conduct some research online to explore the impact of food on inflammation, as many are astonished by the powerful influence of certain nutritious foods on overall health and disease prevention. While the industry often promotes increased vitamin C intake and calorie reduction, it's essential to identify foods that may seem healthy but are not. Recognizing these foods is a crucial step before commencing your anti-inflammatory diet.

Do baked goods feature on your food list? If so, chances are they contain at least small amounts of trans fats, particularly if they are pre-packaged. Even seemingly healthy options like 100-calorie cupcake bites may harbor up to 0.5 grams of trans fats. Consuming just two of these petite cakes daily for a week can accumulate a substantial 7 grams of trans fats, far exceeding the recommended level of zero grams.

Have you been enjoying salads this week? Many people perceive salads as a healthier choice, even when laden with fatty dressings. A mere tablespoon of daily salad dressing can contribute 100 calories and approximately 10 grams of fat, a sizeable portion given that the average serving size is around $^1/\square$ cup per salad. This equates to 400 calories, 40 grams of fat, and an inflammation factor rating of -76, which assesses the food's overall inflammatory impact on the body. The goal is to reach a rating of +50 or higher.

Although few people view food as an adversary, it is vital to understand that numerous life-threatening illnesses are linked to inflammation. Opting for foods devoid of trans fats and low in total fats is a secure means of enhancing your anti-inflammatory response. These adjustments are straightforward, making the diet accessible to everyone.

Foods that undermine the anti-inflammatory diet include pre-packaged items, oil blends, and margarine. Additionally, reducing protein and water intake can hinder the effectiveness of the anti-inflammatory diet. Pre-packaged foods often contain excessive sodium, with a typical meal providing between 700 and 1,000 calories. Consuming these meals several times a week can result in an additional 3,000 calories, along with increased fat and sodium intake. High-fat foods provoke hours of inflammation in the body, leading to weight gain and heightened inflammation. While oil blends are budget-friendly alternatives to pure olive oil, some may include oils containing trans fats. Trans fats are detrimental to health and should be avoided in any diet.

Margarine, though lower in cost and calories than butter, is not necessarily a healthier option. Those concerned about butter's cholesterol content need not worry, as individuals who consume low-carbohydrate diets with significant butter intake exhibit lower cholesterol levels compared to margarine or low-fat consumers.

For those who encounter budget constraints, it may be tempting to substitute lean beef with fatty burgers, which can lead to an increased cancer risk and inflammation. In such cases, it's advisable to opt for beans instead. Water, often described as the elixir of life, is the top choice for improving well-being and reducing inflammation. Some individuals on an anti-inflammatory diet initially consume half a gallon or more of water daily. However, with time, this habit may wane, leading to increased caffeine consumption and reduced water intake. Caffeine can contribute to inflammation and counteract the anti-inflammatory diet's goals.

It's important to note that the anti-inflammatory diet does not necessitate the complete avoidance of all foods that may cause inflammation. Deprivation often leads people to abandon new diets in favor of their previous eating habits. Instead of depriving yourself, consider healthy alternatives and eliminate pre-packaged foods, red fatty meats, and trans fats from your diet. The occasional indulgence is not a problem; the real issue arises when inflammation becomes a recurring occurrence, undermining the benefits of the anti-inflammatory diet, even if you believe you're following it.

Closing thoughts

In conclusion, "The Complete Anti-Inflammatory Diet Cookbook for Beginners" offers a practical and accessible guide to improving your health through dietary choices. This book provides valuable insights into the anti-inflammatory diet and empowers readers to make positive changes in their lives. By offering straightforward recipes and helpful tips, it enables beginners to embark on a journey toward better well-being. Emphasizing the importance of food choices, the book demonstrates how simple dietary changes can have a profound impact on reducing inflammation and promoting longevity. With this cookbook, you have the tools to embrace a healthier lifestyle and savor delicious meals that support your overall health. Start your anti-inflammatory diet journey today and discover the positive transformation it can bring to your life.

9 798862 967654